D0814667

Be Sick Well

A Healthy Approach to Chronic Illness

Jeff Kane, M.D.

Forward by Larry Dossey, M.D.

NEW HARBINGER PUBLICATIONS, INC.

Library of Congress Catalog Card Number: 91-52889

ISBN 1-879237-08-3 Paperback
ISBN 1-879237-09-1 Cloth

Cover design by SHELBY DESIGNS & ILLUSTRATES

Printed on recycled paper

First printing July 1991, 7,500 copies

Table of Contents

For Ronnie Paul
and our daughters,
Alix and Tashie

Foreword

Be Sick Well is a remarkably caring, gentle, and wise book about the human condition, and it is a distinct honor for me to recommend it. It is urgently needed — for, as Dr. Kane points out, most of us will develop, sooner or later, some type of chronic illness: it is only a matter of time.

Today we are learning more than ever before about the role of consciousness in health. We know that our attitudes, beliefs, and choices play a vital role in the development of many acute and chronic illnesses. Some people, however, have taken this to mean that, since the mind is important, it is *all*-important. Some maintain, in fact, that we "create our own reality, 100 percent!" Many people are heavily influenced by this view, and when they become ill they may interpret their illness as evidence of some sort of ethical or moral failure. This problem is particularly vexing for those who develop a chronic illness. This point of view is one of the greatest excesses of the consciousness-and-health movement. It has led to immense emotional pain and has spawned an epidemic of "new age guilt," which begins in the individual the moment things go wrong. Dr. Kane addresses this issue head-on, showing that illness and pain are a natural part of life; that life paradoxically can be made richer by them; that we would lose our ability to feel life if we abolished discomfort entirely; and that spiritual giants develop illnesses just as do spiritual weaklings.

This book is a treasure chest of "what to do" and "how to be" during a chronic illness. It is long overdue. Most physicians do not enjoy dealing with "chronics"; we are at our best when employing spectacular, short-term interventions. That's why this book will be of great value to an immense number of individuals who may feel neglected by the medical establishment, and will assist physicians and health care providers as well. In fact, the book can be read with immense benefit by everyone, even the healthy.

Be Sick Well is a beautiful example of clear, concise communication. This is no accident, for Dr. Kane is a master communicator who is well known for his work in the field of patient-physician interaction.

Susan Sontag once called illness "the night side of life." It *is* a dark moment for everyone — but it also is a *natural* side of life, for day without night has no meaning. Our task is to understand it — to catch its messages, its meanings. To learn, as Dr. Kane tells us, to be sick well.

Larry Dossey, M.D.
Santa Fe, New Mexico
Author: *Meaning & Medicine*
Recovering the Soul
Beyond Illness
Space, Time & Medicine

Preface

Fifteen years and a life ago, I was Chief Physician in a metropolitan emergency department. One spring morning at seven o'clock I reported for a twelve-hour shift.

I changed into a green scrub suit. Loose as it obviously was, it chafed. Nothing else was right, either. The ward's rooms and corridors looked alien, as though colors or materials had been switched. The machinery — the EKGs, defibrillators, surgical kits — that had seemed awesomely powerful the day before now appeared coldly lifeless. I couldn't stay! I asked another doctor to fill in for me, drove to my home in the woods, and sat staring for weeks.

I had wanted to be a doctor since the age of six, when my pediatrician soothed my raw throat instantly simply by touching me. This struck me as supremely useful magic which I became determined to learn. I graduated from college a certified scientist, and a remarkable whisper still reminded me that healing was a discipline of wonder.

My naiveté crumbled on day one of medical training, as I discovered that training would be a long, tough tour of atoms and molecules, biochemistry and physiology, tissues and organs. There was never a mention of the word "healing," let alone a course in it.

I repressed my disappointment for a decade, practicing medicine in a wide variety of settings, from the genteel National Institutes of Health to rough-and-tumble county hospitals. But my original fascination continued to smolder, and ultimately ignited my abrupt exit from the Emergency Department.

Sitting alone in the woods, I came to realize that I'd been competently trained in disease, but hadn't the foggiest vision of health. If you had asked me, I could have recited numerous metabolic pathways and acid-base formulas, but couldn't tell you what constituted a normal human being. With these colossal holes in my little black bag, I was expected to help people — not tissues and organs, but people. I'd aimed to be a priest, a shaman, a healer, and discovered myself to be a biochemical engineer.

I began to see sick people again, but in a different way. I asked them to tell me what it was like to be sick. Uniformly delighted to oblige, these people became the professors of my postgraduate education. Some explained their experience in adequate depth and detail for me to feel what they felt. The more I listened, the more I heard. The more I heard, the more their stories made sense: there were bridges of meaning between their illnesses and their lives.

My new focus on meaning brought me nose-to-nose with the most significant — and most monumentally ignored — issue in medicine, the body-mind relationship. The subject is totally ignored in medical training, the tacit assumption being that the mind is an illusion generated by brain biochemistry.

But I could no longer dismiss the body-mind relationship so perfunctorily. I found a suitable means of exploring it, the venerable Indian body-mind science, hatha yoga.

Yoga is far more than pretzel-like contortions. It offers healing tools useful in daily American life, such as profound relaxation and pain control. On a deeper but less tangible level, yoga students experience internal revelations that steadily expand their lives. The paramount skill — beyond physical flexibility — is the existential stretch: a well-developed person can appreciate a chronic illness as serious business and simultaneously as an opportunity for growth.

I'm closer now to the model of physicianhood that I originally sought. The magic I'd longed for isn't in my little black bag, and can never be. It's in people. May you, the reader, find your share of magic.

Acknowledgments

I hardly ever read authors' acknowledgments since I never know the people the author is thanking.

But sometimes the causes for gratitude are as important as the identities of the benefactors. Emotional sustenance is the foundation upon which a new idea — like *Be Sick Well* — is built. It would have collapsed had those I trusted not encouraged me.

For decades of unquestioning support, I'm deeply grateful to my parents, Herb and Rena Kane.

Beyond mere thanks: my wife, Ronnie Paul, whose love surpasses all understanding.

I thank those who have cleared the path and borne the light, including Elisabeth Kübler-Ross, Ivan Illich, James Creighton, Carl Simonton, Stephanie M. Simonton, Lawrence LeShan, Norman Cousins, Jerry Jampolsky, Larry Dossey, Bernie Siegel, and the other intrepid thinkers who personify a new approach to healing.

I thank my gently incisive editors, Barbara Quick and Patrick Fanning, who regularly guided me from exotica into plainly intelligible communication.

Special thanks go to those who inspired the book by living its ideas — the scores of people who unstintingly told me the stories of their illnesses, often reaching into deeply intimate recesses they hadn't revealed even to their own spouses. I've changed people's names, sexes, and ages here and there to protect privacy, and occasionally aggregated case histories to make a point; but otherwise the stories are true.

1

A Healthy Approach to Chronic Illness

What This Book Is About

This book is as much about you as about your illness.

You must already be aware that the two of you are inextricably involved anyway. In the twenty-four years of my practice, I have never seen an illness jump up onto the examining table all by itself. It is universally in the company of a person.

Undoubtedly your illness has affected you deeply. *The idea of this book is for you to affect your illness through creative rather than passive participation.* If you consider this book's ideas seriously and perform the exercises diligently, you will learn a healthy approach to your chronic illness — which is to say, to your life. Your approach will be characterized by

- An attitude that continually dictates therapeutic behavior

- A degree of confident control over your illness

- Your illness being easier on your family and vice-versa

- Getting what you need from those who help you

- Intense support and love

• The ability to undergo significant life changes creatively

The Significance of Chronic Illness

A chronic illness, as the name implies, is one that stretches out over time. Year by year, it insidiously changes the way you live, the way you think, and, ultimately, who you are.

There's a distinction between chronic illness and acute illness, which usually ends in less than a month (examples are colds, minor injuries, and infections that respond to antibiotics). Some acute illnesses have a way of becoming chronic. A heart attack, for example, can heal partially, leaving behind a case of chronic coronary artery insufficiency (*angina*) or chronic congestive heart failure.

A century ago the most common serious diseases were acute ones, usually infections. People who contracted scarlet fever, diphtheria, and smallpox either died summarily or recovered. Now, with improved nutrition and public health practices, we're living longer — long enough to develop the kind of diseases incubated by aging tissues and declining resistance. Currently the most common serious diseases are cancer and cardiovascular disorders, both largely chronic.

If you live long enough, you will probably develop a chronic disease: cancer, pulmonary disease, arthritis, Parkinsonism, and so on. I take no glee in saying this. I only want to remind you that flesh, like all things, inevitably decays and dies: *chronic illness is part of a normal process.*

The Importance of a Positive Perspective

Seen in this light, chronic illness is not exclusively catastrophic. Dr. Elisabeth Kübler-Ross' work with people who are dying, for example, shows that the palpable prospect of death can generate a powerful appreciation for life, which in turn can elevate the quality of the remaining quantity.

Something similar can be said for chronic illness. If you see your illness as pure tragedy, you'll gain nothing from it but depression. If, however, you see it as an important challenge that demands a creative response, you can act accordingly.

Jack is a thirty-year-old cabinetmaker. He has his own show on a community radio station devoted to education about disabled people. Jack was left paraplegic as a teenager during a motorcycle race. He says, "If it weren't for that accident, I'm sure I'd still be a punk."

This perceptual shift is not easy, for your chronic illness pervades your life as thoroughly as an unwelcome but powerfully tenacious guest. Perhaps your doctor advised you to learn to live with your illness, little suspecting how thoroughly you'd do just that. Whether you wanted to or not, you have literally incorporated your illness: it has united with your body. This being the case, you'd do well to examine all the effects your illness has upon you.

As it constricts your capabilities, chronic illness does no less than change your self-image and your personality. And long-term pain doesn't just hurt — it's exhausting as well. It can be likened to a wide-open energy spigot. Nor does exhaustion stop with you: when you're unable to function optimally, family members have to take up your slack. Unanticipated, tedious responsibilities can generate elaborately braided systems of guilt, resentment, depression, and anger, all of which can exacerbate your illness. Never mind whether these changes are good or bad — they're significant and deserve your attention.

I wish that development of positive attitudes were simply a matter of verbal affirmation, but it's not that easy. For one thing, many people doubt that it's possible. For example, some of your friends believe that a positive perspective is air-brained wishful thinking, that you should leave the matter in the hands of experts and avoid getting involved. Other fragile souls are threatened by any kind of change, whether it's news of your illness or news of steps you've taken to heal it. They may snicker openly about your healing quest. They may whisper to each other that your illness has baked your brain. They may mercifully have the courtesy to leave the subject taboo. This is a complex problem, for while your friends and relations love you and mean well, their negative beliefs will nonetheless thwart your progress.

A creative perspective is not at all wishful thinking, but rather an honest appraisal of the entire situation. This includes the adverse effects of your illness, the resources available to you

— and through you — and the opportunities inherent in any crisis.

> Ryan, a thirty-three-year-old skiing instructor, dramatically began to lose his form. A medical examination revealed he had amyotrophic lateral sclerosis ("ALS" or "Lou Gehrig's disease"), a condition characterized by muscle weakness. At first devastated, he gradually saw his illness as a chance to return to an earlier interest, writing. He has since become a successful freelance writer, focusing on disabled sports events.

Falsehoods About Chronic Illness

So you will need to deal with negative and pessimistic beliefs about your illness. What thickens the plot is that these beliefs are often held by people you trust, including family members, friends, and doctors. I'll list a few such beliefs here to forewarn you. Since they disagree with mine, I'll call them "falsehoods."

Falsehood 1: "You're a victim of cancer/arthritis/stroke."

Don't let anyone whittle your already-threatened self-image down to an icon of impotence, the innocent victim of a hostile universe. Granted you're sick, but you remain a unique human being with a full complement of strengths, needs, and dignity. You are in any case a participant, never a passive bystander.

> Lisa, a thirty-eight-year-old woman with marked rheumatoid arthritis, was so disabled by pain that she had to be turned in bed by caretakers. Her main complaint, though — more than her pain — was her sense of helplessness and loss of control. She was particularly bothered by being at the mercy of one caretaker who she felt was unnecessarily rough. She suffered as a victim until she got angry enough to announce, "You're fired!" The next day she told a gentler caretaker, "You know what? I don't hurt so much today!"

Falsehood 2: "You'll be sick for the rest of your life."

No one knows that statement to be true. Virtually every disease has examples — however rare — of remissions. Remissions are instances of the diseases simply picking up and leaving. When this occurs following medical treatment, we doctors call it a "cure." When it occurs outside medical treatment we call it a "spontaneous remission," which is an elaborate way of saying we haven't the vaguest idea why it occurred. (People who have experienced spontaneous remissions, by the way, uniformly take exception to the word spontaneous. They credit themselves, their families, God, radical change, prayer, and so on, feeling that some kind of deliberate intervention produced the remission.)

The only indisputable thing that can be said about the duration of your illness is that you have it now. As far as the future is concerned, the disease can go any which way, period. It's important to appreciate this notion, for all the suggestions I'll make in this book are based on focusing your attention on the present and not grabbing for any particular future.

Falsehood 3: "There's no effective treatment for your illness."

The bad news is that medical science is fairly helpless in the face of most chronic illnesses. Though our treatment can minimize symptoms or slow a disease's progress, it will not usually cure it.

The good news is that the only limitations we're talking about here *are* the medical ones. In a wider arena, much can be done. As long as you have your conscious mind, you can renovate your attitudes, improve your relationships, garner support, and make changes that elevate your life's quality. Isn't that what you're after in the long run anyway?

Millie, a sixty-two-year-old woman with advanced metastatic breast cancer, decided that she could provide herself more peace of mind by "finishing old business," as she put it. She talked in great and candid detail at her bedside with her son and her ex-husband, clearing up matters that had long been on her mind.

Afterward she said, "Now I can die in peace," and she did.

Falsehood 4: *"You have a life expectancy of six to twelve months."*

Alright, let's talk statistics. All medical predictions are based on statistics, distillations of data from large numbers of patients. What we tend to forget is that by definition *statistics refer only to groups, never to individuals.* When applied to individuals, they are only tendencies that can be grossly misleading. For example, valid data indicate that since more people are alive today than have ever died, you are statistically likely to live forever!

Here's my statistical rule of thumb: three out of four statistics are unreliable, and one out of four is dangerous.

Statistics are unreliable in their poor qualitative resolution: they measure only a limited number of dimensions. Diagnosis, of course, is an important category. So too are age, sex, race, and socioeconomic status. But how often do statisticians take into account diet, relationships, support, stress management, spiritual practices, exercise, and other facets of lifestyle that might bear on outcome? In other words, the only completely reliable statistic about you is the one that simultaneously appreciates every category of your entire life! At that refined level it's no longer a probability — it's your unique biography. So please don't take any statistic as your future carved in granite.

At worst, statistics are dangerous when they become self-fulfilling prophecies. Ask yourself: do people "given" six months die after six months because the prophecy was accurate or because it parasitized their attention? Was the statistic a description of the real world or a subtle prescription for unconscious behavior?

Incidentally, patients often come away from the medical transaction with wholly different data than what they've been given. Few doctors these days make statements as stark as, "You've got six months." When pressed, they might say something like, "Studies show that eighty out of one hundred people with your kind of cancer live six months, and sixty live one year." Patients unused to statistics personalize this into, "The doc gave me six months to a year."

No matter what numbers you come across, keep in mind that at least one other person with your disease has enjoyed a remission. Why shouldn't this be your lot as well?

Falsehood 5: "Your condition is terminal."

As long as I'm on my high horse here, let me trample the notion that you can know when someone is dying. The only way to determine if a condition is terminal is if the person dies. Then you can say with complete certainty that the condition was terminal. In my rasher days — when I felt compelled to predict the moment of death — I was wrong more often than right. I've seen people robust on Monday and dead on Tuesday, and I've also seen people with nine toes in the grave rebound into normal lives.

There's still another way to regard this issue. Consider that until your eventual death you are leading a life, no matter how attenuated it may be.

> Roberta was a thirty-six-year-old woman bedridden with cancer for five years. Her doctors had expected her to die momentarily dozens of times. She joked with me once that the latest tests revealed "...that I have only six normal cells left."
>
> Roberta phoned me one night to complain that she was bored. "Look," she said, "I've been lying around dying for years now. Am I gonna die or what?"
>
> I'd never faced a situation like this before. Flying by the seat of my pants, I responded, "Beats me. Maybe what you have here is one of the world's more unusual lifestyles. I mean that maybe this is just the way your life is going."
>
> "Oh, yeah," she agreed. "I guess if I'd been dying, I'd be dead by now." She dropped her boredom immediately, returned to her usual routine of reading and listening to music, and died peacefully six months later.

Kübler-Ross handles this issue by informing people that they are "seriously ill." That's honest. She has no way of knowing if they'll die from this disease. When patients ask me, "Will I die?", we often develop a wonderful conversation in which they accept that they will indeed die, though not necessarily during this illness. And until they actually die, they live, as do we all.

If you're seriously ill, of course you should take care of your business in this world. Indeed, everyone should, and the best time to do it is before you get sick — as soon as you recognize that life itself is a terminal condition.

Silence: The Indispensible Skill

To regard your chronic illness as a newly revealed path instead of a cruel detour from some "correct" path is to envision a slightly different personality for yourself! This prospect is the opportunity of a lifetime and at the same time possibly the most difficult thing you will ever face.

What makes it so hard is your present personality's tenacity. It insists on stability. So does mine, as a matter of fact. Something inside all of us resists every measly change.

Think of what proportion of your daily life is habitual. Usually people tell me upwards of eighty percent. The phrase has become a platitude, but we actually are creatures of habit. Some clever people define "ego" or social personality as the sum of all habits. We are, in other words, what we do. To change behavior, then, is to change no less than who we are. Threatened to the core, the ego screams, "Don't do it, or...." and follows with a plausible threat: you'll go nuts, you'll join a cult, you'll make a fool of yourself, you'll end up in a snake pit. As the champion of stasis, the mind dredges up whatever it needs to keep you from changing.

This internal dialogue, constantly reinforcing habitual perception and consequent behavior, is called "chatter." You might recognize it if I tell you that Hindus call it "the drunken monkey." Your mind relentlessly reiterates its own point of view. It says that the world is friendly or hostile, that women or men love or hate you, that your kids are wonderful prodigies or intolerable brats, and so on. Never mind what's "really" true. We behave as though our mental projections *were* true.

Doris, a sixty-year-old woman, is chronically depressed. "Why shouldn't I be?" she asks. "Have you looked around? Everyone's depressed. Just go out onto the sidewalk and open your eyes. People look like the end of the world is coming tomorrow. That's what makes me feel so down."

If you agree that your chronic illness presents the opportunity to challenge and amend a few habits, you need to know that you can't change who you are and still remain the same. Something's gotta give. A famous Buddhist story has a zen roshi pouring tea into the cup of a skeptical student until it overflows. He explains, "One cannot fill a cup that is already full."

The skill indispensible to the ideas in this book is the occasional realization of *internal silence*. That mental dialogue, that constant reminder of who you presently are, regularly needs temporary shelving. Turn it off. You can call this "getting quiet," "meditation," "prayer," "autohypnosis," or "relaxation." The label doesn't matter. The essential component of this practice is that the drunken monkey sits still while you confidently experience yourself without chatter. Emptying your cup allows it to be refilled, and often this "new tea" is more useful than the cold, stale stuff.

I suggest that you read no more than one chapter of this book daily, and afterward perform the exercise at the end of the chapter. The exercise may be difficult at first — not only hard, but confusing or even somewhat scary, especially if it's new to you. But stick with it anyway, just as you would need to do if you were learning pullups or endurance running. I guarantee that it will get easier and more familiar with practice.

Exercise: Quieting Your Mind

1. Assure yourself silent, uninterruptible privacy. Turn off the oven, unplug the phone, advise your family, and lock your door. Place an unobtrusive timer under a pillow in your room, set for ten minutes.

2. Sit or lie in a perfectly comfortable position, defined as a position that requires as little physical effort as possible. Any subtle holding or imbalance steals an increment of the attention you're

trying to focus. If you're a novice at this, sit up, as lying down can seduce you into sleep.

3. Watch your breath. Yes, it's as simple as this — and as difficult. Don't breathe any particular way. This is actually an exercise for attention, not breathing. So let your breath come and go in its own natural rate, rhythm, and style. Relax progressively until all you're doing is sensing your breath. Release tension in your limbs, pelvis, abdomen, chest, neck, and face. If you're unsure whether muscles are contracted or not, deliberately contract and then relax them.

Stop fidgeting. All those adjustments, itches, and twitches are chatter. Recognize them and instead of giving in, pretend to breathe around them.

Now notice every aspect of your breath: the air's temperature, humidity, aromas; the passage of air through your nose, around the back of your palate, down your windpipe; the movement of your ribcage and abdomen; the durations of inspiration and expiration; the ease of breathing and consistency of cycles; the relative symmetry of all movement; and so on. If you add an additional aspect with each breath, soon your attention will be so filled with sensation that there will be no room for chatter. The only thing you will experience is the breath.

4. Be persistent, but extremely gentle with yourself. Your mind will chatter almost uncontrollably at first. It will inform you of fascinating new itches, the sound of a bathroom flooding, your IRS audit ten years ago. It will plan you a dinner one evening next July. It can be heavy-handed: "Stop this or you'll die!" It can be cunning: "Congratulations! You've finally quieted your mind!" That is, it will bring up anything necessary to stop you from quieting it.

Don't get angry at your mind. Chatter, after all, is your mind's *modus operandi*. Respond to any and all chatter, *regardless of content*, in exactly the same way: notice it dispassionately and return your attention to your breath. Pretend your breath is a stream that has come upon a boulder in its path, chatter. The stream doesn't try to push the boulder out of its way. It simply flows around it.

5. When your timer signals the end of the session, spend one additional minute to make a graceful transition from your inner, quiet world to the outer world. Don't simply jump back into your daily life, eager for your comfortable old routine.

Despite any contrary assumptions you might have made, you have quieted your mind, however slightly. You may even have allowed one or two obsolete habits of thought to evaporate from your repertoire. As you leave your sanctuary and plug in the phone again, consider that your world might henceforth look just a bit different.

2

Disease and Illness

Sickness, Disease, and Illness

Your illness is your own unique, personal experience.

As such, it begs your understanding, for it holds clues to both feeling better and reshaping your life.

To my way of thinking, the most useful notion to arise within the medical world in the past decade is that *sickness is composed of objective and subjective aspects*. Until now I've used the words "sickness," "illness," and "disease" interchangeably. But now consider these new meanings:

Sickness: The entire process, composed of "disease" and "illness." If sickness were a coin, disease and illness would be "heads" and "tails."

Disease: The physical, objective, measurable aspect of sickness. This is what doctors are trained to diagnose and treat. It includes, for example, how many degrees of fever, pounds of weight loss, extent of swelling, and so on.

Illness: Your subjective, *unmeasurable* experience of the disease; the sum of your suffering.

The distinction between disease and illness is the most important idea in this book. If all you remember from these pages a year from now is a clear concept of their difference, I'll feel fulfilled.

I can express the idea's significance best by saying what might at first sound blasphemous: *Cancer never bothered anyone.*

There, I've said it. Cancer (arthritis/lupus/migraines/whatever) never bothered anyone.

An irreverent statement, but true. What bothers people with cancer, for example, is not the tumor or any disorder of function, but their own experience of it: fear, pain, guilt, depression, anxiety, despair, and so on. If the disease didn't exist, neither would the illness — but that doesn't mean they're the same. Illness and disease are two clearly different aspects of a single phenomenon.

> Robert, a professional yoga teacher, sought medical help for lingering neck pain. X-rays disclosed severe arthritis. "My doctor couldn't understand why I was so upset by 'a little arthritis.' He began to tell me what treatment he planned to keep it under control, but I couldn't hear a word he said. What kept running through my mind was that I'd never again be able to do headstands — that my career was ended."

Illness as Your Own Experience

Occasionally I ask an audience, "Who here has had the worst pain?" A few people tentatively raise their hands but sheepishly drop them upon realizing that the question is silly, unanswerable. There's simply no quantitative way to compare anyone else's feelings to your own.

That, after all, is part of what we mean by "subjective": permanently unmeasurable. Further, there will never be an objective "pain meter" simply because such measurement necessarily involves a subjective report. Something as sophisticated as a polygraph — a lie detector — monitors such functions as skin wetness and breathing rate; but its measurements are obviously not identical to whatever the person subjectively experiences.

Christine, a fifty-year-old woman, was furious about what her doctor told her. "She couldn't find a cause for my headaches. She's ruled out migraines and tumors and God knows what, and now she says there are no physical reasons for me to have these headaches, so they're 'all in my mind.' But I have them! Does this mean I'm a psycho?"

In other words, your subjective experience — your illness — while admittedly unmeasurable, is *real* and therefore deserves your full credence.

But we doctors have lacked effective methods for addressing illness.

We approach disease with a powerful model, pathology, which holds that all diseases can be traced to objectively verifiable changes in human structure and function.

The pathology model requires a search for the diagnosis, the correct name of the disease process. In standard practice the doctor takes a history, performs a physical examination, develops a "differential diagnosis" — a list of plausible possibilities — and then requests the laboratory tests and other procedures needed to zero in on the correct diagnosis. Once secured, the diagnosis dictates both the treatment and the prognosis, which is a prediction of the disease's course.

This pattern is internally consistent and actually quite potent toward its own end, the treatment of disease; but it characteristically leaves the patient's anguish — the illness — unaddressed. The commonly recognized medical mission, the diagnosis and treatment of disease, is often pursued without much attention to the alleviation of suffering.

Before our modern secular era, many people looked to the clergy for the alleviation of their mental and spiritual anguish. But as popular faith shifted in this century from religion to science, the doctor began to be perceived in the role of priest. This shift would have served us well were we doctors trained in priestly arts. But, for the most part, we are not: subjectivity is all but excised from medical training. Those rare physicians who deal with their patients' experiences as well as their diseases have developed this skill on their own initiative.

Think, then, of medicine as half of an effective partnership. You've hired your doctor to deal with your disease. But it's up to you to deal with your illness. Note that dealing with illness is not at all an "alternative" treatment, but a necessary complement to standard medicine.

Generally speaking, the more you participate, the less your doctor will need to intervene. The reverse is true as well: the less you address your illness, the more your doctor will need to treat your disease.

> Jack, fifty-seven, has been hospitalized six times for breathing difficulties stemming from his emphysema. He says, "I tell my doctor, 'Doc, you just do what you need to do and I'll go along with it. I'll leave it entirely to you.'" Most of the day Jack is connected to a breathing machine via his tracheostomy. He spends much of his machine-free time in the visitors' lounge, smoking.
>
> *   *   *
>
> Ellen suffers from chronic pulmonary hypertension. "I just hated to carry around that portable oxygen gadget," she admits, "so I paid better attention to when my breathing became more difficult. Wonder of wonders, it was when I was under stress. A respiratory therapist showed me how I unconsciously hampered my breathing when I got upset — I tightened my chest, neck, and belly without even thinking about it. She showed me how to relax even when things get tough, and now I don't need the machine as much as I did."

So how can you address your illness? By ending your cigaret habit? By learning more effective breathing? Yes, and more. I described earlier the route your doctor takes and now I'll describe your parallel assignment.

Illness as a Story

Illness, a process that is by definition unmeasurable, is difficult to elucidate. But if we were to have a model analogous to pathology for describing illness, we would be able to examine both sides of the coin instead of just the physical one.

For many of us who work with illness, a model has begun to emerge: *illness is like a story*. This story can be to illness what pathology is to disease.

This notion ought to fit just about everybody's experience. You love to tell stories, don't you? You don't go through life believing yourself to be a billiard ball at the utterly random mercy of other balls and cue sticks. I assume that you've told others about your illness — what you're going through — as fully as you related your last vacation.

Further, I'll bet your story has gradually evolved. Do you remember how you described your illness at first? What happened to your story as you repeated it over time? It changed, didn't it?

Our personal stories change with time. These changes tend to be greatest early on. Essential elements persist and are polished, while less essential and less desired elements fade away. Over months and years, as the teller fine-tunes the tale, it becomes more stable. At last it becomes eligible for admission to his or her portfolio of personal myths.

"I got polio right after we got married," says Art. "It was a shock because Connie thought she'd married this athlete, this huge, supple hunk, and now she's left with a guy in a wheelchair...."

Connie interrupts: "Art, you didn't get polio after we were married. You got sick a full year before. I knew what I was getting. When will you believe that I didn't marry you for your body?"

"Well," Art answers, "you know, I've never felt right about being this way with you..."

* * *

Andrea has had chronic leukemia for the past five years. Before then her life was no bed of roses, either. She'd been through two divorces, one of her four children was in jail for drunk driving, and another died of a drug overdose. She's interpreted every adverse event as proof of the universe's malevolence. She was convinced that her leukemia fit this picture perfectly.

While driving to a doctor's appointment, her car was sideswiped by another vehicle. Although Andrea was unhurt in the accident, her doctor determined that her leukemia had worsened. "That was the last straw," says Andrea. "That woman who hit my car destroyed the last of my resistance. If I die from leukemia, it's her fault. I've already asked my lawyer to draw up the papers to sue her."

As a myth, your story needn't be "really" true, since it's actually a composite of real events, fancied memories, and wishful thinking that combine to make sense in the largest possible view — which is to say both in the "real" world and within your imagination.

Even though your life may not be fully comprehensible, you make sure that your stories are. If you're anything like me, as a matter of fact, your own stories so fascinate you that you generally behave not in response to "real" life itself, but in response to your interpretation of it. A poet once said, "Poetry is a lie that makes us see the truth."

A few weeks after surgery for a noncancerous brain tumor, Pearl had a striking dream. "I dreamed I jumped out of an airplane with a parachute," she says. "At the proper time, I pulled the ripcord. But the parachute didn't open. The ripcord broke and just came off in my hand. So there I was, free-falling ten thousand feet toward certain death. I turned the ripcord over and over in my hand, staring at it. I'd never seen such a fascinating braid...."

"I never thought much about my dreams before I got sick," Pearl observes, "but now I seek help everywhere. I interpreted that dream as a message about learning from every experience. Since then, I haven't been as angry about the tumor. I'm not wild about it, but I've been able to see the background as well as the foreground. I've especially noticed how many people love me."

"Illness-as-a-story" is a means by which you can understand how your illness "fits" within your life and, consequently, what will constitute your most positive, powerful response. So do yourself a favor by discovering your story and then telling it in the most positive way you can.

Discovering Your Story With an Illness Journal

I've noticed many times that my thoughts were at best unclear until I spoke them, wrote them down, painted, or in some other way expressed them. My revealed thoughts often surprised me. For this reason I believe an "illness journal" to be an elegant tool.

An illness journal is nothing more than a notebook in which you record the results of exercises in this book, relevant observations, and any ideas that come to you.

> Fred, a thirty-five-year-old physician, fractured his pelvis in a bicycle accident. Two weeks later, he wrote in his journal, "I fell right on my beeper [medical call device], which got driven into my hip. Totally smashed the beeper." He wrote that the injury literally "slowed my pace," something he'd been aiming toward for several years but somehow hadn't been able to bring about. He added, "I guess the smashed beeper tells me something, too."

In addition, I suggest that every week you write a brief encapsulation of your whole story. Periodically thumb back to see how the story has changed.

> Ruth was troubled by her lower back the past year, having initially injured it while lifting something heavy. It never totally healed, so she decided to keep an illness journal. "The story has changed a great deal," she says. "My first entry simply describes the injury. A month later I wrote that it felt like three separate injuries, as though I'd been pulled apart in three directions. Last month I wrote that my three directions seem to be my role as wife, my role as mother, and my own role in the world. I'm beginning to think that

what I need to do is to integrate these roles into a single identity."

Remain steadfastly cognizant that your illness — your personal, subjective experience of this sickness — is as important and at least as treatable as the disease for which your doctor is seeing you. Regard your illness as an event, however painful, that you can squeeze a lesson from.

> Odette has chronic eczema on her hands. She's been seeing the same dermatologist for twelve years now. "He's been wonderful," she exclaims. "He has never once put me down, no matter how wild my ideas. Last year I wondered aloud to him whether my rash was so much worse under my wedding ring because I was having problems with my husband. He laughed and said maybe I was right, and that if I didn't straighten out things at home, he'd give me a new medicine. Well, I told him last month we'd straightened things out and I wouldn't be needing any medicine."

I suspect that the world is actually a Rohrschach test, that events are inkblots upon which we project very personal meanings. Affecting your life as it does, illness is an inkblot that's difficult to ignore. So you will manufacture its significance, its meaning, from the raw material of your mind. That is, your story of your illness is essentially a reflection of your personality.

> Forty-year-old Kevin had lumbar disc surgery ten years ago and never made a complete recovery. He couldn't accept that he still hurt and was partially disabled. "This can't happen to me," he constantly told his wife.
> His original story about his injury was simply that he had been in great shape and was inexplicably struck down; but over time he saw that his illness included his relationships with others. "I always thought of myself as Superman," he says now. "Not just the strength, but, well, the righteousness. I couldn't stand to watch any kind of wrongdoing. Truth, justice, and the American Way were my personal responsibility. Hardly a day went by when I didn't change someone's

tire or break up a fight. I guess I just saddled myself
with unreal expectations."

As Kevin has deliberately declined to right the
world's wrongs over the past year — not an easy
change for him — his back has begun to heal.

* * *

Richard's amyotrophic lateral sclerosis (ALS — "Lou
Gehrig's Disease") increasingly weakened his body.
A brilliant mathematician, Richard was fascinated by
the idea that ALS doesn't affect the head. "That's just
like me," he observed. "I've always lived in my head."
All who know Richard agreed; in fact, the wasting of
his body seemed to stimulate his already impressive
intellect.

Considering his condition further, Richard con-
cluded that his body plays a role in his story as well.
"ALS has paralyzed me, but that's not really a new
situation," he says. "I realize I've always been am-
bivalent about everything, as though my brain wants
to do one thing and my body another. I can't ever
decide which way to act, so I leave myself kind of
paralyzed."

So far Richard has not chosen to change this pattern. When asked how he feels about his ambivalence,
he good-naturedly responds, "Oh, so-so."

Richard's wife is less than enthusiastic about his assessment, and has accused him of claiming to have
created his ALS. "No, I don't believe I created it," he
answers. "I don't know where it came from. This is
just my way of making it make sense"

Tell your story as it comes to you. The way you choose to
express yourself is a personal power that transcends all physical
degradation.

Jim steadily lost weight and stamina with every oppor-
tunistic AIDS infection. But he always kept his spirits
up, his friends say. "He was sure he'd beat it early
on," says one. "He laughed more than ever. We could
rely on him to be the life of the party. When he wasn't

partying, though, he looked depressed. I asked him about it, but he'd flip on a happy face and just deny being depressed. The last dance we went to together, he told me he realized his destiny was to be the first sick AIDS patient to make a permanent recovery. The night he died he told me he felt great. He was sure he was on his way back to good health. I think he was denying a bunch of stuff all along. And I'm not willing to say that was the wrong thing for him to do."

Even if you believe that you can't change your life, you can always change your story. This shift — in your imagination, in your perceived possibilities — can also change your life.

Henry, who had what he describes as a frightfully repressive childhood, thought only about women. His fantasies were old-fashioned and pleasantly romantic. They didn't affect his daily functioning, but he felt unable to daydream about anything else. So for most of his life Henry feared he was neurotic. "I didn't make any headway with my first two therapists," says Henry. "They told me I might have a permanent obsession."

Henry acquired a new therapist who, having heard Henry's history, asked, "So what's the problem?" Surprised that this therapist missed the obvious, Henry responded, "Well that's abnormal! Isn't it?"

"It's certainly unusual," said the therapist, "but I ask you again: what's the problem?"

The therapist asked Henry to consider that he may well be normal and perhaps even gifted. Henry was soon able to trust this notion. To this day his life is productive, and he continues — happily now — to fantasize almost exclusively about women.

* * *

Mike has been paraplegic since his spine was severed in a traffic accident ten years ago. When asked about his condition, he usually replied that "an accident wrecked my body." Calling himself an "invalid," he lived as though his life stopped when he was injured. He characteristically remained at home, depressed.

A paraplegic friend finally coerced Mike into visiting an independent living center on a day when a group of developmentally disabled children visited. Mike suddenly saw dozens of people with arguably greater disabilities than his own. One retarded ten-year-old jovially asked Mike, "So what's wrong witcha legs?" Surprising himself, Mike laughed and answered, "Nothing's wrong with my legs. They just don't work." "Oh," said the kid, satisfied, and walked off.

Mike has volunteered regularly at the center since then. He's also become married and employed.

Be easy on yourself. Keep in mind that not everyone needs to approach their sickness as I recommend in this book; standard medical treatment alone may suffice. If a story is to come at all, it will come without strain. Digging for the story of your illness can get to be a palpable stress. At that point, your frustration actually becomes part of your illness — and this is a complication you don't need. If this happens to you, do what numerous religions around the world suggest: give up. Throw in the towel. Surrender. That's when things sometimes change.

Cecille, fifty-one, had an uncomfortably sizeable but benign thyroid nodule that she and her doctor were watching. Familiar with the disease/illness distinction, she was anxious to develop a story of her illness. For weeks she wrote observations in her journal and waited expectantly for dreams, but was unable to weave a coherent story. One morning she told her husband, "I just don't know what I'm going to do!" She wrung her hands and finally burst into tears. "I give up!" she cried. "It's just a goddam thing in my thyroid, and it doesn't mean a thing!"

That night she dreamed that she was about to sing to her friends. When she opened her mouth, no voice came forth because of a lump in her throat. The lump ascended and popped from Cecille's mouth as an egg. Curious, she cracked it. A full-grown, iridescent pheasant emerged, kissed her, and flew up to the clouds. The next morning Cecille wrote in her journal, "An egg? A kissing pheasant? I have no idea what all this means, but at least I have some stuff to work with now."

* * *

A surgeon removed half of Ray's cancerous left lung a year ago. "I had a complete exam six months ago and again last week," he says, "and the docs have given me a clean bill of health. I feel fine. I think it's kind of weird when people talk about 'learning from their illness.' I don't think there was anything for me to learn. I had cancer, it was caught in time, and now I feel fine."

Ah, but how flat life would be without these stories! It is myth — not objective reality — that drives our lives and inspires us to transcend our present limits. Try reading this true story, for example, without finding meaning in it:

Chet and Linda were married 49 years when Linda got breast cancer that rapidly spread to her brain. Asked why he insisted on accompanying Linda into the examining room during office visits, Chet answered, "Whatever she's got, I've got."

When Linda finally sank into a coma in the hospital, Chet held her hand all day and night. At five o'clock the next morning Chet left the hospital to get breakfast. While he was away, Linda died.

True to their routine, the nurses removed Linda's jewelry for safekeeping. But they couldn't get her wedding ring off, even with lubricants. Mentioning nothing of the jewelry, the nurses gently told Chet that Linda had died while he was gone. He asked for a few minutes alone with her. When he emerged from the drawn curtains, he held the wedding ring in his palm.

Curing and Healing

Why should you address your illness as well as your disease? Do you expect that by dealing with your life you will cure your cancer? *Will resolution of an illness cure a disease?*

The answer, both "yes" and "no," requires that we clarify what "curing" and "healing" are. If you recognize the difference between disease and illness, you'll see the crucial distinction between curing and healing.

With proper medical intervention, I can kill the bacteria responsible for your strep throat, for example, or surgically remove a colonic polyp, and consequently cure the disease.

But as a story, illness cannot be cured. Whatever the story is, it's only a story. There's nothing to cure because nothing is "wrong": *it's perfectly normal to experience the emotions that constitute illness.* That illness is normal, however, doesn't mean it's comfortable. When ill, we yearn for comfort and peace; we yearn all the more when the disease seems permanent or terminal.

Healing, then, is progress toward serenity. With this in mind, you can heal yourself even when your disease is relentless.

> Six-year-old Bill developed a kidney cancer that didn't respond to medical treatment. Like any parents, Ralph and Bernice were crushed. Bill, though, through his discomfort, felt differently. "Won't I be going home to God?" he asked his parents, repeating what they'd always taught him. To the astonishment of his family and the hospital staff, Bill cherished this vision until he died. "It was Billy's faith that kept us all together," recalls Bernice. "Billy taught me more in his few years than I'd learned in my whole life."

> * * *

> "How is it?" I asked Roger, a hard-driving business-man dying from leukemia. "It's like a rough cross-country flight," he joked. "Rough weather, cardboard food, some nausea, and God only knows who's going to meet me at the terminal. It's a good thing I've handled this before." Bringing his extensive travel experience to this final journey, Roger was able to tune

out some of his discomfort, put up with much, ask for help from his numerous "flight attendants," comfort his family with his confidence, and die peacefully.

Healing your illness may well influence the course of your disease. We've known clearly for decades how hopelessness and helplessness wreck people's immune responses. You don't need tablets carved in stone by a presidential blue-ribbon commission to know intuitively that all else equal, you'll do objectively better with a positive outlook than with a depressing one.

> Ginny broke her wrist while "playing" with her boyfriend. Though set and casted properly, the break refused to heal. Her orthopedist planned to pin the bones together.
>
> A nurse, Ginny imagined the injured area as crowded with bone fragments and other anatomical structures. "There are veins and nerves and tendons crawling all over each other..." She paused. "I guess it looks like a jungle; the structures are all vines and such. It's dark. It's dangerous in there."
>
> On reflection, Ginny realized that she viewed her world as a jungle, where the apparently friendly can be hazardous. "Well, that's what I learned from my parents," she admitted. She came to see that she typically behaved with her boyfriend and others in a stiff, flinching manner, as though she expected the worst, and that her injury resulted from inflexibility born of her inherent fear.
>
> "I don't need this anymore," she said. Recognizing fearfulness as obsolete in her current world, Ginny experimented with pretending that the world was a kinder place than she had assumed. Under the influence of this new image and attitude, the bones went on to knit uneventfully.

It's important that you aim your work at your illness, not at your disease. This is a difficult point. When I see seriously sick people individually, I emphasize that our work will illuminate them personally: but that the course of their disease, though related, is a separate matter. By now I'm no longer surprised when, during the second or third session, they ask, "How come I'm still sick?"

Would Ginny have established her more positive attitudes if she were certain that her bones would *not* knit as a result of her efforts? Would you? What reason is there *not* to move toward serenity, with or without being sick?

For a different perspective on this point, consider the practice of running. Some people run to forestall a heart attack. You can tell which ones they are because they are grim runners indeed. Others look like they're having a good time; they run because it jolly well feels good. In other words, an act that to one person is a flight from death is to another a joyous activity. So if you're going to address your illness, do it for immediately present benefits, not for future potential. Your personal efforts can indeed influence your longevity; but to enact them for that reason alone is like running to evade the Reaper, forgetting the joy of the activity itself.

Besides, attitudinal changes are all we're sure you *can* affect. That's certainly more than we doctors can guarantee from our work. As clever and effective as we like to think we are, we can only apply our knowledge and hope for the best. Along with Mexican *curanderos* and African witch doctors, Western physicians must recognize that our craft is threaded with elements of chance, miracles, and fallibility.

You may need to remind yourself repeatedly that curing and healing are distinct endeavors. This perspective may help: diseases are cured, but people are healed.

Harry retired seven years ago from his position as an English professor at a highly regarded university. Two years ago he developed lymphoma that responded at first to chemotherapy but lately has become more intractable. Through discussions, journal-keeping, and an active support group, he's learned much.

At a support group meeting a member asked Harry why he seemed so obviously agitated. "I've been exploring myself and my lymphoma for a year now," he growled. "I've learned a lot. I've made some changes. But I still have the goddamned thing!"

Clara, another group member who has cancer, gently responded, "Harry, wouldn't you have wanted to make those changes anyway? Haven't they improved your life? Besides, how do you know that if you hadn't done this kind of work you wouldn't be dead now?"

I can't improve upon Clara's comments, but I can offer a few additional tips.

Consider your illness an opportunity to achieve deeper self-understanding. Do so and I guarantee success. I also guarantee that if you act upon your understanding you will raise the quality of your life.

Don't be afraid to use your sickness as an all-purpose excuse. You've earned it. Since sickness pulls you off the playing field and plops you onto the sidelines, you might as well use the time and distance to review and renovate your attitudes. That is, take advantage of the situation: *you may now have your "druthers."* If you don't want to drag yourself to Uncle Max's dreadful annual barbecue or if you can't bear the thought of your twisted school chum's impending visit, just say no, you're sick. See what it's like to have things your way, but ask yourself continually, "Can I arrange in the future to have my 'druthers' without the excuse of my sickness?"

Come to terms with your mortality. This isn't as simple as buttering a bagel. It may seem terribly daunting at first, but, like anything you've ever feared, this won't be as threatening once you begin. At least think about it, whether or not you're sick now. Discussing your own mortality with others, especially with people who can handle the subject, will give you a greater perspective, if not calm most of your fears.

This assignment is germane because when I last checked the figures, the ultimate mortality rate was still stuck at 100 percent. Death is a certainty, and its universal cause is life. You might outrun the Reaper today, but he'll always be waiting to shake your hand at the finishline. This doesn't mean that you've lost, just that your race is run. Death isn't a defeat any more than arrival on this planet was a victory.

Exercise: Storytelling as a Way To Transform Your Illness

This exercise will help you make a story of your illness through careful exploration of a symptom. Symptoms are defined as physical feelings that are in some way unpleasant and from which you seek relief. I'm sure that you can describe a pain, for example; but can you appreciate it as a part of your life and actually tease a little meaning from it?

The challenge in this exercise is to translate a symptom into an image. With proper guidance, you can arrive at a juicy, voluntarily generated "dream" which is as fully interpretable as any unconsciously generated dream. To orient yourself, consider first the following examples.

Jose, a middle-aged man with six grown children, developed tenderness and pain in the muscles of his thigh for no apparent reason. His doctor diagnosed the problem as "fibromyositis," an inflammation of unknown cause. Over six months Jose tried several drugs, among which only steroids seemed to work. Pessimistic about remaining on this potentially hazardous medication, Jose decided to attend to his illness as well as his disease.

Focusing intensely on his thigh pain, he described it as a "gnawing" feeling. "It's as though a giant cat is chewing it," he said, surprised at the image's ferocity. In his mind's eye, Jose shrank the cat to kitten size and converted it to an imaginary, innocuous terrycloth doll. With this maneuver, his pain stopped dramatically for the next twenty-four hours.

Jose's unconscious choice of images baffled him until his wife Elena suggested that the cat might represent the Kit-Kat Club, a cocktail lounge where his youngest daughter, Rosa, worked. Rosa left her husband two months ago and moved back in with her parents. Having Rosa home again was far from smooth. Jose admitted, "You know, I'd like to kick her out." Elena responded, half-joking, "With which leg?"

Jose suddenly made the connection: he hadn't realized before how angry he was with Rosa. He and Rosa had an intimate, if heated, talk that night, and she moved out the next weekend.

"We both felt better after clearing the air," recalls Jose, "and I was able to sleep without pain for the first night in a long time. At this point I still hurt some, but at least my doctor's taken me off steroids."

* * *

Terry is a forty-year-old, self-employed graphic artist who had surgery a year ago for ovarian cancer. Recently her doctor discovered a new tumor within her pelvis.

She decided to supplement medical treatment by meeting with me to explore her illness. She focused her attention in her slightly distended abdomen. "It feels like something filling me," she said, "something expanding into a vacant area." Over a couple of sessions she refined her description to "the filling of a void."

She wrote in her journal, "I'm beginning to understand this tumor as a little 'friend' being made for me. I wonder if my 'void' is a lack of friends." She looked at her life and discovered what her acquaintances already knew: she was not a warm person. Indeed, Terry assiduously avoided close relationships during her entire life.

She eventually decided that her cancer held this message: "You cannot continue as you have. Change or die." Although she regarded a change of this magnitude to be supremely threatening, she pursued it anyway. Over the next several months she became strikingly and sincerely outgoing. Her sister said, "She's absolutely fun to be around now. It's as if the old Terry died and a new one took over."

The tumor shrank. Terry returned to her career. Her physician congratulated her: "You're enjoying a spontaneous remission!" Terry answered, "Nothing of the sort — it wasn't spontaneous at all. I did it."

1. Assure yourself a half-hour of quiet solitude. I hope this is becoming an established routine that's getting easier. Before you

begin the exercise, select a symptom you'd like to explore. *Don't start with a serious or life-threatening symptom like severe difficulty in breathing or the feeling of an abnormal heart rhythm.* We learn to walk before we run, right? So start with a minor pain or even an itch. As you develop your skill you can confront more serious symptoms.

2. Quiet your body and mind as you've learned to do in the previous chapter.

3. Also as in the previous chapter, place all your attention in your breath. Fill your attention with every imaginable aspect of the breath at once. Then breathe into the area of your symptom. We both know that you're not really pulling air into, say, your belly — you're pulling attention into it, using the breath as the vehicle. Pretend that every inhalation concentrates attention in the symptom and every exhalation releases whatever attention remains in unrelated areas.

4. Treat the symptom with cautious respect. Approach it the way you'd approach a porcupine: spiral in toward the center from the periphery. The idea is to *appreciate the symptom purely as a sensation devoid of emotional ornament.* Note if your first reaction upon noticing the symptom is something like, "Ow, it hurts! I don't want it to hurt!" or "What a macho dude I am for taking this pain!" Both such reactions are distracting chatter (what I just called "emotional ornament"), and not representative of the symptom itself. If this happens, back off and try again with even more careful respect.

5. Once you feel that you can appreciate the symptom purely as a sensation, begin to characterize it metaphorically. What does it *feel like*? I usually run imaginary flash cards through my mind, comparing the sensation to many others I've experienced or imagined. Is the pain a little like a knife? What kind of knife? Paring knife? Bowie knife? Saracen scimitar? As you retain your attention in the symptom, work toward refining the metaphor. What does it feel more like? A lot like? *Exactly* like? You want to come to such a thorough and accurate description of the symptom that someone hearing your description would feel what you are feeling. That is, be a consummate poet.

6. Since the symptom is by definition unpleasant, the image into which it's accurately translated will exhibit unpleasant features as well. Find these features.

> John's taking an inward look at his chronic low back pain. "It feels like rope," he thinks. But that makes no sense to him. How does rope hurt? He explores his image. "It's the twist in the rope," he remarks to himself. "It's a 'twisting' kind of pain. It feels just like the way nautical rope is twisted."

7. Change your image into an ideal image. Keep in mind that the image is of your own creation, entirely under your control. Change it by any means within your imagination. Keep changing it until it's what you would call "perfect," as ideal and pleasant as you can imagine. Don't hesitate to use methods that seem silly, impossible, or illicit. Persist. If the first method doesn't work, invent another. In the world of imagination, everything is fair and possible.

> Lorraine is an English professor who was having great difficulty preparing her students' final exam. Every time she sat at her desk to do it, her right eye developed an involuntary spastic twitch. She'd noticed this symptom over several years now, always when she was under pressure.
>
> She relaxed and placed her undivided attention in the muscles that operate her right eye. Immediately she saw a vivid image, a nasty green little man "...with a black derby and five o'clock shadow." The imaginary demon had grabbed the opposite ends of an extraocular muscle, and was jerking them together, making her eye twitch.
>
> "First I made myself as tiny as he," Lorraine said. "I tried to reason with him. But he was angry and really mean. I couldn't reason with him. I pleaded with him. I told him how important my work was. He couldn't have cared less. Finally I made myself a lot bigger and just hauled off and punched him in the nose...."

"Then I could see the muscle and the eye clearly. The muscle was still a little pale and taut, so I pinked it up. Pretty soon everything looked as good as new.

"That exercise stopped the twitch right away. But I'd never known before how angry I was, and how my difficulty in getting the exam together wasn't just a coincidence. If the little man hadn't been green, as a matter of fact, he'd have looked a lot like my department chairman."

8. Return your attention to your daily world. As soon as you can, *record the exercise* in your illness journal. What symptom did you explore? What did it feel like (the metaphorical image)? What was unpleasant in the image (what seemed to represent the symptom)? How did you change the image? What was your final "ideal" image?

In changing the image into a pleasant one you will often stop the symptom dramatically. Occasionally, as with a minor symptom, this relief is permanent. Sometimes the symptom will persist or it will disappear and return; and then it becomes worthwhile to explore it for meaning.

9. Interpret the image. By means of the exercise, you've converted an unpleasant physical sensation into what is essentially a dream picture. Most people agree that dreams are elegantly encoded, interpretable messages about the self.

The most important interpreter for your dream is you. After all, the images are your own. So first record your interpretation in your illness journal.

You may be blind, however, to your own images simply because you are so accustomed to them. For this reason you may find it helpful to ask someone else's opinion. So share these "dreams" with a good listener: your spouse, friend, relative, minister, or therapist. Record their interpretations. Keep in mind that your interpreters have their own unique imaginations. What they offer are valuable hints and flavors; but no one has the "objective" truth about your subjective world. Ultimately, the most useful meaning is the one with which you feel most comfortable.

3

Illness and Attitude

Attitude

You may not have control over the physical, objective aspect of your sickness, but you can always influence your outlook. In this chapter I'll suggest methods of achieving a healthy outlook, or what I call a *therapeutic attitude*.

Since your illness is defined as the emotions that accompany your disease, treatment consists of feeling, understanding, expressing, and in all ways coming to terms with those emotions appropriately. Ideally, your illness is healed when you experience serenity in the presence of your disease.

Emotions are expressions of attitude, and attitude is changeable.

"When Sally was seven," recalls Sally's mother, Liz, "she got leukemia. The first few times we brought her in for treatment, she was terrified. She laid awake the whole night before, too scared to sleep. By the time her doctor saw her she was a nervous wreck, and it wasn't much better for us, either. Fortunately, the hospital had a child counseling team that had seen this before. They accepted her in a part-time program that was like a

school, and some of what the kids learned was how
medicine, doctors, and hospitals helped kids, even
though the help was sometimes painful. Gradually
Sally began to accept her treatments as part of her life.
She returned to her normal sleeping habits and really
became more curious than frightened. She's twenty
now, completely cured, and in her first year of medical
school."

But attitudinal change is serious business, for an attitude is
more than what you say it is. If you're familiar with the notion
of "body language," you know that the mouth and the rest of the
body can give different messages.

Kathy, twenty-two, married Ted two years ago. During
that time her rheumatoid arthritis flared more often
than ever before. Frequently her pain forced her to can-
cel social plans she and Ted had made, so they stayed
home. She read, he sulked.
    She said, "Ted, is everything okay?" "Sure," he
muttered. Kathy got the message — Ted was angry
over social deprivation — and she began to feel guilty.
At the same time, she was angry at Ted's reaction because she felt justified in canceling their plans. So she
sulked.
    They barely talked to each other for two days.
Finally Ted asked, "So what's wrong with you?"
"Nothing," she replied.

He says everything's okay and she says nothing's wrong. I
hope you don't believe what they say. Sulkers can't possibly be
having a good time. This we know: the mouth knows how to lie
but, unless you're an actor, the body — the organ of behavior —
does not. *How you describe your attitude, then, is inconsequential compared to how you enact it.*

Composed of emotional experiences, illnesses exhibit rather
predictable phases which I categorize as acute, subacute, and
chronic. Each phase requires a slightly different healing strategy.

Acute Phase: The Confetti Syndrome

The "acute" phase of a chronic illness comes and goes relatively quickly. This phase usually occurs from initial realization of the sickness until a few weeks afterward, although I've seen it as short as two days and as long as several months. Consisting of tremendous emotional intensity, mood swings, and disorientation, this is illness' most uncomfortable period.

I call this the Confetti Syndrome because the unwelcome diagnostic news figuratively shreds your stable life and tosses it into the air, and all you can do is wait for the pieces to fall back into some comprehensible picture. After all, the onset of a chronic illness places your life at an unknown crossroad. I would be surprised if you didn't feel shocked, confused, and helpless in this alien landscape.

A healing attitude requires that you know a few important things about the Confetti Syndrome.

It is normal. There's nothing weird or neurotic about feeling disorganized or literally scared out of your wits upon learning that your life may change willy-nilly or that you're potentially facing death. Sickness is difficult enough, so I advise you not to worry about your sanity as well. In the midst of the chaos you might forget you're normal — so ask friends and relatives to remind you.

The exact manifestation of the syndrome is idiosyncratic, unique to every individual. That is, you may encounter bursts of virtually any emotion and even many together. Some people feel the Confetti Syndrome as an emotional roller coaster. Expect surprises. Whenever I think I've seen it all, I come across something new.

Marian, a thirty-five-year-old mother of two small children, learned that her chest pain was not bronchitis, but a particularly malignant cancer. The next day she giddily said, "You know, I'm not depressed like I thought I might have been. I'm actually kind of elated. At last I've got the opportunity to clean all the crap out of my life!"

* * *

Dan, a middle-aged executive, learned that he had
colonic cancer during a routine company physical. He
agreed to the surgery appointment his doctor made for
the following week. Although he had no symptoms
whatsoever, Dan didn't go to work before his surgery.
He stayed in his basement, played with his model
electric trains — a hobby he'd ignored for years — and
ate continually. Dan's diagnosis and planned surgery
didn't disturb his wife, Rhonda, as much as Dan's
strange behavior did. She'd ask, "Dan, are you okay?"
"Sure I'm okay," he'd say, "but would you bring me
another sandwich please?" "Alright, Dan, but don't
you feel like going to work?" "No, not today. I'd
rather stay down here."

A therapist friend who visited with Dan later in
the week reassured Rhonda that Dan was reacting normally in a situation where "normalcy" has particularly
wide boundaries. He went through his surgery successfully, recovered uneventfully, and returned to work and
his normal diet.

It is meaningful. The Confetti Syndrome is your innate
healing drive shifting into action. You are sculpting yourself a
new self-image. If you feel like your very personality is coming
unglued, you're right. Whoever you were before the diagnosis
has already metaphorically died. And while your previous self-
image is gone, you don't have a good handle on your new one
yet. But it is on the way.

The whole process is a potentially therapeutic renovation
that requires disintegration before reconstruction. You've heard
the proverb, "To make an omelet you need to break eggs." The
Confetti Syndrome is the period right before the omelet, except
that there are broken shells on the floor and yolks on the walls.
It's hard to believe now that this mess could transform into something even remotely pleasant or useful. But a few intrepid folks
have preceded you, so the process isn't entirely mysterious. Consider this period as an invisible bridge between who you were
and who you will soon be.

It is not time to act. Friends will phone, visit, and write
with suggestions, advice, information. They may avalanche you

with stacks of articles and books they want you to read. Forget it. Do nothing. You can't read, listen, or even think attentively now anyway.

It's especially important that you make no significant decisions while the confetti's up in the air. There's hardly any course of treatment that won't wait until you gather your wits.

This is a frustrating time for those who want to help: for the best thing they can do now is what you should do — nothing. Nothing, that is, about your illness. If folks really want to help, ask them to cover some of your daily chores so you can devote more attention to going through this period more gracefully.

> "My doctor just sat me down and matter-of-factly told me I had lymphoma," says Estelle. "I've worked in doctors' offices, so I know what lymphoma is. Then he told me what he was going to do about it. He went on and on. I wanted to say, 'Stop! Don't you know I've heard all I can, and can't hear more?' I thanked him and went home.
>
> "I live alone. I just sat for three days and stared. I have no idea what was on my mind. A few friends found out, and then the news got around quickly. My best friend, Bonnie, took charge and told people that I didn't need all their cures now, I needed their physical help. I still cry when I think of all the food they brought, how they cleaned my house...."

It is finite. It will end. You can hasten the confetti's fall with the application of your skills and the support of others.

> Jack lost his hand in a factory accident. His wife, Rosemary, was alarmed that he sat in his rocking chair and simply rocked, day after day. He spoke with Rosemary in monosyllables and barely recognized visitors. The factory medical office called in a visiting nurse, a gruffly warm woman named Nellie. Taking one look at Jack, Nellie asked his visitors to leave. "He's not ready for visitors," she announced. "He's not ready for anything except rocking." Nellie let Jack know that he was reacting normally to a catastrophic event, that he was sure to come out of it in his own

time, and she'd love to listen anytime he'd like to talk.
He soon talked plenty, and screamed and cried as well.
Two weeks later Jack began to joke about his disability
and invited friends in. "He became like a new man!"
says Rosemary. Eventually he was fitted with a pros-
thesis and returned to work.

It can recur. Sometimes a disease will progress in stepwise
fashion despite the most effective known treatments. Just when
you think your life has stabilized, the disease tosses the confetti
into the air once again.

But you've seen this before, so at least it begins to become
familiar. A comparable pattern is adolescence, which, with its
rapid changes, carries an almost daily need for adjustment of self-
image. One thing that people with progressive diseases learn —
just as members of Alcoholics Anonymous learn — is to live each
day for itself, one day at a time.

Tom, fifty-three, has been diabetic since childhood. "It
was hard as a kid," he recalls, "sticking my finger, test-
ing my blood, and giving myself insulin; but it was
especially hard being different. I got used to it the best
I could, though.

"I began to have eye troubles at twenty because of
diabetes. When my doctor got me lined up for a guide
dog I panicked for a month. I realized I was going
blind! Well, I did go blind. That hasn't been easy, but
I've managed.

"I've had a great marriage and enjoyed my career.
Things were going alright. But last year my left toes
got gangrenous because of the diabetes. After they
were amputated, I mainly slept for a couple of days. I
didn't even know I was depressed, I guess, but then it
became obvious for a couple of weeks. But I got over it.

"Now I'm having trouble further up the leg. I've
accepted a diabetic and insulin lifestyle, blindness, and
now I'm looking at the prospect of being whittled
away. Maybe I've gotten used to shocks like these. I
don't like them, but I'd never have been able to face
this now if I hadn't known the earlier ones."

Subacute Phase: Intense, Discrete Emotions

A "subacute" process lies between an immediate, acute one and a chronic process of long duration. Occurring after the Confetti Syndrome, the subacute phase lasts anywhere from weeks to months.

You'll know the confetti period is behind you when your emotional tornado resolves into a steadily distinguishable emotion you can name, such as depression, anger, fear, or anxiety. Yesterday you would have said to yourself, "I'm sick and also crazy/disoriented/confused/desperate," but today's message would be, "I'm sick and I'm anxious." For better or worse, you're off the roller coaster. Welcome back.

Now is the time to act. There's much you can do toward achieving a healing attitude. To be exact, you can move toward accepting your disease.

I'll need to put this suggestion delicately, for it is as important as it is outrageous. I know you don't want to be sick. Perhaps you're angry about it. Or you're sad about it, say, or desperate. But remember: these emotions are precisely what constitute your illness. Imagine what your disease would feel like if you sensed it purely, without emotional decoration. It's not easy, of course, but if you actually can — *if you can be sick without feeling one way or the other about it* — *you have healed your illness.*

You've accepted your disease (or treated your illness — these are one and the same) when you have dealt effectively with all the emotions that comprise this subacute period. It's to be hoped that you'll finish being depressed over your disease. You'll drop your anger about it. As you come exclusively to appreciate the present, you'll harbor neither hope nor hopelessness. In terms of what I said earlier about words versus body language, it means that you will become as relaxed as possible in the presence of your disease.

I know this will bring up a few issues for you, so here are some answers in advance.

You don't have to like your disease in order to accept it.

Sam suffered a stroke that left his right arm immobile. At first he was depressed about the loss, and even spoke angrily to his own arm on occasion. But he proceeded with physical therapy anyway. After six months, he simply stopped being angry and told his wife, "I don't see any improvement in it. I guess I'll just go on without a right arm." Sam became an expert lefty, even to the extent of writing and one-armed golf.

* * *

Fred was furious at the world about his cancer. "How can you say there's a God when stuff like this goes on? Why do I get it and the President of South Africa doesn't?" Fred spoke like this almost constantly. Eventually his doctor diagnosed an ulcer in addition to the cancer, and advised Fred to learn to relax. "How can I relax," Fred asked, "when good people drop like flies while those crooks in Washington get richer every day?"

Fred's wife, Karla, finally got tired of Fred's complaints and warned him that she was going to leave if he didn't shut up. This caught his attention. He took several deep relaxation workshops. "You know," he confided to Karla afterward, "I have a lot more energy now." "Of course," she said. "You're putting your outrage calories into more positive stuff."

When he felt up to it, Fred did volunteer work with troubled teenagers and usually came home tired but fulfilled. He gradually sickened, though, and when I asked him on his deathbed, "Fred, how is this for you?" he grinned weakly and replied, "Matter of fact, it's not so bad."

Acceptance is not the same as pessimistic resignation to your disease. On the other hand, it doesn't necessarily mean that you'll be cured of it. In short, acceptance has nothing to do with the future: it's simply an acknowledgment of the incontrovertible present.

Millie, a meditation teacher, developed severe arthritis in her lower spine. She suffered constant pain in her back and down both legs. "I took all kinds of medicines for a year," she recalls. "They helped some, but they had pretty bad side effects. I couldn't go on like that. But I didn't want to give in to the arthritis, either.

"I really thought about it. All along I had this feeling I was fighting against the arthritis, like it was some kind of war going on inside my body. I finally figured I was really fighting against myself. So I decided on an approach closer to my meditation practice. I began to meditate on my pain.

"This was scary at first, because I thought that concentrating on the symptom might make it worse. But I did it anyway. Talk about 'accepting' my illness: I climbed right into it! The more I meditated on my pain, the more it seemed to recede into the distance. I found that this approach gave me terrific control of the pain. I don't know if I've controlled the arthritis because I haven't had x-rays for two years now. Actually, I don't even care how the arthritis is. I don't hurt."

Give yourself time. Lingering depression can represent real grief for the loss of your former self-image. How long should this take? Don't assume that it "ought" to take three days or four years. Even though we know we can shorten its duration with adequate expression and support, grief takes as long as it takes. It's amazing what people can accept if they take the time for accommodation.

Tim was a superb athlete. A husky six-foot bodybuilder and runner, he often decried those who fell out of shape or became sick. "Jeez, if I was like that," he said once, pointing to a man with a limp, "I'd slit my wrists."

A broken neck from a diving accident paralyzed Tim's legs, partly paralyzed his arms, and sent him into a profound depressive tailspin. More than one doctor recommended that his family institutionalize him. But after a year he began to insist on caring for himself, using a variety of aids and a motorized wheelchair. His sense of humor returned. Passing another quadriplegic on the street, he remarked to his friend,

"Jeez, you see that guy drooling? If I was like that, I'd slit my wrists."

Chronic Phase: Recurrent Discrete Emotions

A chronic process is a long-term one. The pattern of the chronic phase describes emotions that recur over a longer period of time. During the subacute period, for example, you may have gone through a depression. Perhaps you handled it as well as anyone could, but, to your frustration, here it is again. *Recurrent emotions that you experience in this phase are less a part of your illness than they are deeper personality traits highlighted by your sickness.*

You will deal with these emotions in the same way you deal with any others; but you should be aware that their duration — their tenacious seniority, if you will — makes them more resistant to modulation or control.

Maude, a remarkably independent eighty-year-old widow, broke her hip in a fall. She underwent corrective surgery successfully and was sent to a convalescent hospital to recover. The nurses noted during the first few days of Maude's stay that she was mildly confused, depressed, and inappropriately angry. But her wit soon returned, and other patients described her as a joy to be with.

Ten days after her surgery, a food service worker informed Maude's nurse that Maude had literally screamed at her about her dessert. When the nurse questioned Maude about it, Maude got furious again and threatened to cane her. Familiar with the medical literature that recommends psychoactive medication for tantrums in older people, the nurse planned to ask Maude's doctor to prescribe a tranquilizer the next morning. But Maude woke up as gentle and friendly as could be, so no steps were taken.

Her son visited that day. The nurse told him about Maude's outbursts. He replied, "Oh, that's Mom, alright! She's always been like that. You just can't tell when she's going to fly off the handle." Knowing this about Maude, the nursing staff acted differently. "We stopped taking it personally," says the nurse, "and treated her as though she didn't mean to be that angry." Maude soon returned home, where she continues to this day to throw occasional temper tantrums.

Guilt

Guilt is the most common example of a recurrent emotion experienced by sick people. It deserves special exploration because of its almost universal association with sickness in our culture.

There's no shortage of guilt. If it were currency, we'd all be rich. And if it were all justified, the world would be an intolerable place. In sum, there's too much *unnecessary* guilt. It's fine to feel remorse when you've done something you knew was wrong. But as often as not, folks feel guilty and can't for the life of them recall what it is they're guilty about.

There's nothing to feel guilty about when you're sick. If you curse yourself in some way for getting sick, reflect that everyone gets sick one time or another, some get sicker than others, and everyone eventually dies. That is, *sickness is a normal feature of life*. So if I were granted a wish, it would be for sick people to mail their guilt to folks who could use a little more, like, say, munitions manufacturers.

Nevertheless, people understandably feel guilty when their sickness affects others. When you're sick you can't function; others must work in your place. Family members who are normally dependent on you must now be your caretakers. Your sickness has disrupted your home, workplace, and social relationships.

Franny developed a progressive spinal arthritis that limited her endurance as a food service worker. The company's medical officer recommended "light duty," a permanent desk job. Consequently, her co-workers had to absorb the work Franny had previously done. This made her feel terrible, a feeling she continually communicated to her colleagues. They soon wearied of her whining. One said, "Look, Franny, we can manage the work. What we have trouble with is listening to your apologies. Any of us can get sick. You're doing your best. If you must feel guilty, please at least keep it to yourself." Franny recalls, "It was then that I realized I had two problems, and the arthritis was probably the lesser of the two."

I suspect that some illness guilt results from the attractive myth that we should all be healthy and live long lives. There is abundant historical precedent behind this myth. In his book *Medical Nemesis*, Ivan Illich points out that an image of death was ubiquitous in medieval art. The skeletal specter attended every feast and wedding. But as modern medicine flexed its early muscles — by the eighteenth century — artists regularly depicted a physician standing between Death and his potential victims. By the nineteenth century, Death had left the picture entirely. In other words, we romanticized the power of medical science. We continue to do so; when you get obviously sick — when you've reminded folks that all is not laughter and glamour — you feel guilty in part because you've broken a taboo.

It amazes me that we send our anthropologists to every exotic cave and jungle while they could be having a field day at home. They would probably advise us that taboos can be useful and they can also become obsolete. When taboos lose their utility, popular practice gradually phases them out. Take heart, for being sick will soon be acceptable again. Trust me. Not so long ago, remember, sex was an unmentionable subject, too.

Blame

Maybe you can deal with the guilt about how your sickness affects others. But here's an even tougher issue: whose fault *is* it that you're sick?

You've probably been taught since childhood that disease strikes unwitting victims, that it's purely impersonal, and you have nothing to do with its inception. Well, take a deep breath and have a seat, for that's not entirely true. We know, for example, that the causes of serious diseases such as cancer and arteriosclerosis include lifestyle elements — diet, exercise, stress management, and toxic exposures — which are largely chosen, either consciously or unconsciously.

This means that you may have *contributed* to your disease by smoking, overeating, or leading the life of a hyperstressed couch potato. This doesn't mean that you caused your disease; "contribution," remember, is not identical to "cause."

Even if you acted unhealthily, sickness occurs in a more complex way than cause-and-effect. Some smokers, after all, *don't* get lung disease, and some chubbies *don't* become hypertensive or diabetic. Conversely, a few of the piously fit come down with diseases that are seemingly reserved for body abusers. Go figure it out if you can.

Whether or not you recognize any personal contribution to your disease, you're involved with it simply by experiencing it. But involvement isn't the same as causality, either. Still, I'm impressed by how often people, on discovering their inevitable involvement, flip suddenly from innocent bystander to Typhoid Mary. It's as though they tell themselves, "If my sickness wasn't handed to me randomly, then I must have created it myself."

Even worse, I've seen well people with the best of intentions lay this blame on sick friends and relations.

Nelda returned home from the hospital after being medically regulated for insulin-dependent diabetes of sudden onset. Her first visitor was Barbara, a friend interested in "new age" healing ideas.

"Nelda," said Barbara, "I want you to get that you created your diabetes because you need more sweetness in your life."

Nelda, who already felt guilty about the diabetes' disruption of her family life, asked, "What do you mean, I 'created' my diabetes?"

"Well," said Barbara, "not consciously, of course."

"If I need sweetness," said Nelda, "why don't you just be sweet to me? Guilt I don't need."

Bravo! More guilt hardly any of us needs, so here are a few tips for laying your burden down.

Forgive your past. I've done more than a few dumb things myself. But now I know better, so I don't create identical idiocies. Also, I can forgive myself for past transgressions because I recognize that I did the best I could at the time. I was more ignorant, insensitive, or preoccupied than I am now. I can choose to suffer guilt from my past errors or choose instead to forgive myself, learn from my mistakes, and try not to repeat them.

> "I've done terrible things," says Milt. "At the time, though, I thought they were good and even noble. When I was a Green Beret I helped wipe out an entire village in Cambodia. Everybody — kids and grandmas and pets — everybody. As the helicopter lifted us out, it felt like a veil came off my eyes. I saw vividly what I'd done, and realized a couple of things. First, I'd done my best, such as my best was at that moment. Second, I decided to use the rest of my life to know better, to know better every day."
>
> Milt immediately resigned his commission, arranged his discharge, traveled to India, and, to shorten a longer story, became a "saddhu," a wandering monk. He made his way to Calcutta, where he cared for dying people in a hospice. Today he counsels dying people in the United States. "I know more about guilt than anyone I know," says Milt. "The only thing anyone should ever feel guilty about is refusing to become more conscious in their life."

Decide that in the future you'll forgive yourself for what you fail to see in your behavior today. Maybe what you do today will look cruel or self-destructive to you ten years from now. But you'll recognize again that you did the best you could considering your present-day, relatively invisible limitations.

> Veronica hated her job because of her poor relationship with her supervisor. She used any excuse she could find to provide herself a "mental health" absence. Having taken all her vacation days and administrative leave, she called in sick, claiming to have a sore throat. She wasn't sick, of course, but as the day wore on she ironically developed a sore throat and by the next morning really was sick.
>
> "So I thought to myself," she muses, "'How would I tell this story a few years from now? Will I say I made myself sick?' And then I thought, 'Why should I

get sick over my supervisor being a jerk? Why take it
out on myself? Never mind whether I really gave myself a sore throat — the issue here is that I'm weaseling
around about my job.'" As she resolved to confront her
supervisor directly, her symptoms mysteriously
vanished.

You'll find it easier to forgive yourself if you forgive others.

"I used to know why everyone got sick," muses Barbara. "This one's lung cancer was held-in screaming.
That one's colitis was her guts crying. My friend Nelda
got diabetes because she needed sweetness in her life. I
thought I saw how everything worked, but I got a
whole new perspective when I learned I had breast
cancer.

"Sickness just happens, period. We can use it to
learn about ourselves and change for the better, but
we'd do well to forget about claiming we caused it.

"If my friends weren't aware of everything in their
lives, neither was I. We're all just doing our best.
Nelda didn't get diabetes in order to make her life
sweeter; she just has it, and I can help her by giving
sweetness. I don't enjoy having cancer, and I didn't create it, but it sure showed me deeper understanding."

Distinguish between "blame" and "responsibility." People
usually confuse these concepts, assuming that responsibility for
an untoward event constitutes blame for it as well. Forget this.
Tape this definition to your refrigerator instead:

"Blame" is liability for a prior event.

*"Responsibility" is the **ability to respond** to a present
situation.*

Picking apart the past is as useless while you're sick as
straining for the future. Concentration on anything except the incontestable fact that you're sick now is a waste of calories.

Frank, a forty-year-old bachelor, admits, "I ate barrels
of saturated fat and hardly ever exercised. I put myself

on a few ascetic diets too grim to maintain. I tried jogging but it just gave me tension headaches. I finally had to look at why I didn't take better care of myself.

"It dawned on me that I'd always treated myself hatefully! That made me angry at my parents for allowing me to grow up like that. But mainly I was furious with myself for letting my body become tapioca. I almost beat my head against the wall one night, but I realized suddenly that all my anguish was taking the form of even more blame and self-hatred. Then I knew I needed help.

"I joined a men's group and learned that these feelings were pretty common. It took awhile, but I began to think of myself more positively. Then I just found myself eating healthier stuff and wanting to exercise. I didn't plan it — it just happened. I'm not tapioca anymore."

Fight or Surrender?

Now that you have a few more tools to promote a therapeutic attitude, how will you use them? Will you gently accept your situation or confront it with a warrior's gusto? Which style works better?

Several respected studies have shown that the chronically sick people who live the longest and enjoy the highest quality in their lives are those who are the worst patients. These "survivors" are ornery, independent people who scoff at hospital regulations, skeptically question doctors' advice, and, from what I've seen, can't wait to throttle the Angel of Death.

You have a little paradox on your hands. You know that feisty folks do better, but on the other hand people like me suggest that you continue to "accept" your sickness. So which should you do, fight or surrender?

Both.

Fight versus surrender is, in fact, a false distinction. Opting exclusively for either will dilute your effort, because fight and surrender are complementary; each is a vitamin for the other. Here's how they can mesh:

To act powerfully, first surrender. Only when you have accepted your sickness — feel relaxed in its presence — can you formulate a realistic fight plan. Short of this, fear and anxiety will generate jagged, half-hearted responses, and you'll waste valuable energy on impossible quests.

> Bill is a strong man, a can-do building contractor, who also has lung cancer. "Sure I'm gonna beat it," he initially told his family and friends. But the cancer spread through his body, greatly weakening him. "Don't worry," he told visitors, "I've always done what I set out to do, and I'm gonna beat this cancer."
>
> One night in the hospital, a morphine-induced dream frightened him enormously. He told a psychiatrist the next morning, "I dreamed I was as tiny as a speck of sand caught up in bulldozer treads. I said I'd get up in the driver's seat, but the bulldozer ignored me. This was the first time I ever experienced something I couldn't handle."
>
> Working with the psychiatrist, Bill came to conclude that one thing inevitably beyond his control was his eventual death. "Right," says Bill now, "but that doesn't mean this cancer's going to get me today. And even if it does get me today, it's not getting me right now, while I'm talking to you." Instead of predicting his certain triumph over cancer, Bill currently speaks of moment-to-moment accomplishments.

To surrender, be powerful. Acceptance of your disease demands that you do the most difficult thing in the world: gain control over your mind.

The mind, remember, constantly reiterates its litany of stability. It resists all change, especially its own demise. So your mind will insist that you'd rather not be sick, you don't want to die, you'd like your old life back, and so on, typically heedless of reality. Universal as it is, this is a kind of mental tail-chasing that cannot but wear you out. "We have met the enemy," said comic-strip character Pogo, "and he is us." Many people have described their illness to me as the most harrowing *and* the most educational adventure of their lives.

At the age of forty-seven, Ruth thought she was going insane. She couldn't believe that menopausal hormone patterns could account for her wild mood swings. One day she'd be full of energy and creative ideas, the next day she'd contemplate suicide. Hormone replacement pills only slightly improved her symptoms, reinforcing her feeling that she was insane as well. One physician who examined her felt that she was manic-depressive, and recommended lithium treatment.

Ruth finally found a psychotherapist who'd recently been through menopause herself, and had suffered similar symptoms and anxieties about the symptoms. This therapist advised Ruth to consider her mood swings not as any sickness, but as a normal albeit irksome process secondary to hormonal change. She affirmed more than once that Ruth was not going crazy.

Now finished with this transition, Ruth says, "The scariest thing about it was the fear that I was losing my mind. That was worse than the mood swings themselves. But my therapist taught me to meditate by watching my worst fears without getting caught up in them. Sure enough, after a while I was able to see that there is a 'me' in addition to my mind.

"Besides raising my kids, that ordeal was the most difficult thing I've ever done. My car now has a bumper sticker that says, 'Pain is inevitable; suffering is optional.'"

Learning From Your Illness

If you read again through the case histories in this chapter, you'll note a common theme: all these people learned extensively from their experiences with sickness. It's reasonable to conjecture that, had their illnesses not occurred, they would not have learned what they did.

Most people who have reaped wisdom from their illness will ask themselves, "I wonder if I could have learned that without getting sick." This naturally generates the next question: "What can I learn *now* without getting sick?"

Linda was a major executive with an insurance company of national reputation. "My work demanded my continual attention," she recalls. "They were certainly paying me enough for it. I couldn't afford to take sick days." She routinely went to work with colds during a harsh winter, but awoke one morning literally unable to get up. "I called my secretary and said I'd be able to work in bed, on the phone. She told me she wouldn't hear of it.

"So I actually took the day off. I laid there thinking all kinds of things, especially about what a wimp I was. But I also felt how really wonderful it was just to rest. Anyway, I returned to work the next day. By nighttime I had a fever and was coughing up pus. My doctor wanted to put me in the hospital. Actually, she was pretty sick herself at the time; I was as concerned about her as she was about me. So here we were, two sick professional women, each demanding the other take care of herself. I got her to let me go home on antibiotics and she kept working.

"The next morning I was still feverish and becoming disoriented, so I called my doctor again. I found out she'd already been hospitalized by her partner. Her partner hospitalized me, too. I had meningitis. Another hour without treatment and I'd probably have died."

Linda spent a week in the hospital and the rest of the month recuperating at home. "One of my job's fringe benefits was excellent medical insurance, so my hospitalization didn't cost me a penny. But I realized when I was convalescing that if my job had benefits, it had hazards, too: part of my terrific salary was for ignoring some of my needs.

"I don't work there anymore, and I now make far less in a job that lets me take care of myself. These days I see even mild fatigue as a message I'd better take seriously."

A comedian once said, "Death is nature's way of telling you to slow down." Is sickness a potential lesson, or is it just a random event or cosmic error? I don't regard disease itself as a vehicle of wisdom, but I do see it clearly as an opportunity for you to discover more of your own inherent wisdom. Of course, that view is only my preference, for there's no way to know what sickness "really" is. You must draw your own conclusions and act accordingly.

Exercise: Drawing Your Illness and Healing

This exercise is to help you discover subtler features of your illness — attitudes raised by your disease — than you have noticed so far. It's different than exercises in other chapters in that it's not meant to be a mind-quieting exercise. On the contrary, it's a mind-stimulating one in which I ask you to push your imagination to the limit.

Compare the lessons your illness has to teach you with the act of fishing. You can sit up on the dock and wait for fish to leap from the water and flop at your feet. Actually, you might get awfully hungry waiting for this to happen.

Alternatively, you can set out a baited line: instead of waiting for ideas to come to you, go searching for them. This exercise is a search. I'll ask you to rummage through your imagination for the answers to these questions: *What constitutes your illness? And what would constitute your healing?*

The only ground rule is to treat this exercise as child's play. That is, resist temptations to criticize your artistic abilities or inhibit your expression.

1. Assure yourself thirty minutes of quiet and privacy with just two sheets of paper (two pages in your illness journal will do nicely) and a set of colored pencils or crayons.

2. Take ten minutes to create an "illness drawing." Draw what your disease means to you. If it were an object, what would it look like? How big? What colors? Is the disease like a dinosaur? An explosion? A raincloud? Or draw what you look like with this disease. Does it make you feel small, wounded, disfigured, abandoned? Include any elements you feel are important. You may or may not want to include family members in your drawing. If all you can draw are stick figures, fine.

This exercise is similar to the one you did at the end of Chapter Two — translating a feeling into a pictorial metaphor.

This time you're extending it from your mind's eye onto paper, ideally creating a picture so emotionally accurate that an outside viewer would feel what you feel.

> Phyllis, who has an unusual form of bone marrow cancer, describes her drawing: "I have a halo and horns, but no ears or facial features. I'm wearing my son's Purple Heart (given to me when I had lung surgery). There is a concealed heart in my belly. My feet point in different directions. My chest area is blue. My arms are green, possibly signifying growth. While my legs seem colorless, my feet are brown."

3. Take ten minutes to create a "healing drawing." What will your healed life look like? Will there be rainbows, unicorns, a quiet pond? Will you look larger, a different color, more at ease? Again, this drawing may or may not have people in it. Note what elements of your drawing seem to represent the healed state. Just as you may have felt sad or anxious while drawing your illness, you may feel lighter as you draw your healing.

> Phyllis describes this second picture: "The halo and horns remain, but I have a face that expresses alertness. I have ears. There's movement throughout my body. A strong red heart is in the right place. Again, there's 'growing' green in my arms and legs. My feet, working together, are ascending steps. My body is filled with light and has a spiritual (blue) aura."

4. In your illness journal, record an interpretive description of each picture, similar to the nature of Phyllis' descriptions above. This step is important because often you're not aware of exactly what you've expressed in one mode (say, in a picture) until you express it in another (say, in words). Then write your impression of the difference between the two pictures. In contrasting your present attitude about your condition with your ideal imaginable attitude, you will begin to comprehend a healing strategy.
Here's how Phyllis did it:

> "The first picture suggests to me that I'm stuck, trying not to show emotions or feel vulnerable. My feet are brown — feet of clay? The second figure looks alive,

flexible, and flowing. Now, which is the real me?

"I am, of course, both. My first picture reminds me how I've been so self-judgmental, sad, unsure, inexpressive. My second picture shows my self-judgment still present, but I'm much warmer, more accepting, flexible. Exercises like this have helped me develop more gentleness toward myself and consequently toward others."

5. As in the exercise in Chapter Two, ask someone you trust to tell you what he or she sees in the two pictures, the differences, and an overall interpretation. Record this information in your journal along with your evaluation of the other person's comments. Do you agree with them or not? Did he or she find themes you missed?

6. Save the drawings as part of your journal. Repeat the exercise in a month. Compare what you learned today with what you discover later.

4

Your Illness
and Other People

A Bomb in Your Living Room

Illness changes habits.

The habits I'm talking about here are the ones people use to relate to each other. Take your family's habits, for example. Let's say you never discuss death with your husband because of the fearful and frightening way he reacted to his mother's painful death. Suppose you automatically get angry whenever the kids come home with a new dirty word. Suppose you routinely give in to your mother's unreasonable demands because you learned early in childhood never to hurt her feelings. You may not be aware that these are habits even as you enact them, but they are habits nonetheless.

Now suppose your husband has contracted a serious illness which begs contemplation of his mortality. How strictly will you avoid the subject? Or your kid has learned a new dirty word while hospitalized for her cystic fibrosis. How mad will you get? Or suppose your mother develops Alzheimer's disease and her demands on you escalate to the tyrannical and nonsensical. How will you respond to her now? In other words, will you question your comfortable, time-honored habits?

These habits are not merely behavioral quirks. They are markers of self-image, defining who you are. A useful way of understanding your social sense of self, or your "ego," is as the sum of all your habits, including those you don't consciously recognize. That is, your habitual patterns of relating to others form a large part of your identity.

So it is that a challenge to your habits is no small business: it shakes the foundation of your personhood. That's why all of us resist every change so vehemently. Dozens of seriously ill people have told me, "Help me, doc! I'll do anything!" This plea often expresses more desperation than motivation, as it soon becomes apparent that many folks will do anything — except, of course, change the most trivial habit.

> Richard saw his doctor because of pain in his head and abdomen. "I hurt all the time," complained Richard. "I can't go on like this. Along with everything else, it's just too much to take. I'm desperate!"
>
> The doctor diagnosed both borderline high blood pressure and an ulcer. He advised Richard, "Your body is telling you that you can't go on like you have been. You're going to have to find some way to move out of the fast track."
>
> Richard agreed to slow down, beginning with learning how to relax. But he didn't get far. "I bought a relaxation instruction tape and listened to it every day, but I just couldn't relax," he admits. "Whenever I tried, I kept repeating to myself all the things I needed to do. Frankly, it seemed like doing my regular stuff was more important than relaxing. So I changed doctors. I need to take a bunch of medicines now and I have a few side effects, but at least I can lead my usual life."

In *On Death and Dying*, Elisabeth Kübler-Ross observes that people confronted with the tangible prospect of their own death undergo a predictable series of emotional acrobatics, including:

Denial: "Not me. They got me mixed up with another patient."

Anger: "Why me? Why not that schmuck who lives down the street?"

Bargaining: "I'll eat my veggies if you'll just give me two more years."

Depression: "Aw, what's the use?"

When these and other reactions have been confronted successfully, what is left is what she calls acceptance, a dispassionate recognition of the situation, a quiet state that's hospitable to the seed of healing.

Kübler-Ross' observations may be validly applied to virtually any major unpleasantness, including auto accidents, job loss, miscarriages, and IRS audits. Take divorce, for example:

Denial: "What!? You're kidding me!"

Anger: "Why, you bastard! I've always known you were carrying on behind my back!"

Bargaining: "C'mon, honey, I promise I'll go on the wagon."

Depression: "No one will ever love me again."

Depression expresses your grief for what you've lost. Again, if you navigate skillfully through these stormy waters, you'll reach the serene island of acceptance, where you comprehend that the change is not necessarily "good" or "bad," but unquestionably is. Whatever the actual situation, this is the point from which you begin to build a new life.

The diagnosis, progression, or recurrence of chronic illness is certain to rock your emotional boat. In fact, I would be shocked if someone with arthritis, cancer, or Parkinsonism seemed unaffected (in fact, I would suspect them of being in denial). Emotional turmoil is a normal feature of chronic illness.

One seldom-described feature of chronic illness is that it's not only you, the sick person, who faces emotional turbulence, but everyone around you as well. Your pattern of social habits has meshed more or less with those of your family, friends, and colleagues. In altering these habits, your illness tosses a monkey wrench into machinery that has been fine-tuned over decades. Everyone close to you goes through a variant of Kübler-Ross' stages:

> *Denial:* "Don't worry about it, Tom. You'll be as good as new next week."

> *Anger:* "Dammit! You would have to throw your back out again just when we have that important tournament coming up!"

> *Bargaining:* "Please, God, if you'll let her walk again I promise to be a better mother."

And, of course, all the people who are close to you will go through depression, even though they're not the ones who are sick. Your friends and relatives grieve not only for your loss, but their own: they miss the part of themselves that has been nurtured by their relationship with you prior to your illness.

I was medically trained in the notion that sickness is nothing more than a misery randomly visited upon innocent individuals. Indeed, we Americans act as though a germ or carcinogen has singled us out from the herd and exclusively marked us for invasion. In anthropological language, we believe sickness to be demonic possession, a personal curse treatable with an exorcism purchased from our white-coated witch doctors.

Obviously, it's not all that simple. Sickness is not an individual phenomenon. It connotes a complex web of profound social effects. *A cancer is not just a tumor; you might understand it better if you think of it as a bomb that's gone off in your living room.* This simple perceptual shift will prepare you to respond most therapeutically to the people in your life.

Your Illness and Your Spouse

Your husband or wife is especially vulnerable to your illness, as he or she is usually what's called your "primary caregiver." That is, the spouse is most likely the one who cooks, cleans, transports, screens visitors, plans functions, and perhaps even washes you and turns you in bed.

Your changes — physical and emotional — mean more to this person than to anyone else, for he or she sees you at your most debilitated while at the same time retaining an ideal image of you. After all, it was your spouse who was charmed enough to want to share life with you.

Romantic notions are no small matter, helping as they do to define reality. Think back, for example, to when you first began to fall in love. Remember how moles became "beauty marks" and wrinkles became "smile lines?" It wasn't the objective world that changed: bumps and creases remain bumps and creases. What changed was what you made of the world. Love polishes everything, and then we behave as though the world were wonderful. Who's to say this magic isn't desirable?

But perhaps effects of your chronic illness have made you diverge from your spouse's romantic image. You may lack the energy she admired. You may develop a facial rash that turns your husband off. Your spouse may react to your dependence with revulsion instead of cheerful service. What has happened here is that your spouse has noticed that he or she can no longer reconcile objective with subjective reality. A major perceptual shift is necessary. *The chronic illness that does not stress a marriage is exceptional.*

It's a platitude to point out that a wife and husband come to look more like sister and brother as years go on. People who live together for decades pervade each other's lives thoroughly, and a chronic illness will predictably follow the lines of interpenetration. Hardly any aspect of the relationship will be unaffected: devotion, dominance, communication habits, sexual relationship, source of income, relationship to children and parents, external friendship needs, and so on.

Consider your spouse's physical difficulties. You can't work, so your wife may need to get a second job. You can't clean the house, so she must do it between when she comes home and when she cooks dinner for you. So in addition to her emotional response to your sickness, she's seriously exhausted as well. Will you be surprised, then, when she begins getting crabby with you? Will you be surprised at your own feelings of guilt?

It's crucial to recognize that the process is not uniformly terrible. Hidden opportunities abound. Because the regular contours of the relationship have deformed, you and your spouse may see things in new ways. You may, say, get a fresh look at your own tendency toward dependency, along with ideas for addressing it creatively. Your spouse may find that old resentments toward you emerge unexpectedly, and can then be free to decide whether she still needs to carry them. You both may find deeper connections with each other. In any case, you will discover features of the relationship that would have remained hidden had the apple cart not tumbled. So here's the bad news: it can be a whole new ball game. And here's the good news: it can be a whole new ball game.

Knowing the hazards, what can you do about it? I can't present a complete tour here of all possible problems and solutions, but here are a few initial hints you may find helpful.

Assume, despite any verbiage to the contrary, that your illness, as a significant event, affects your marriage deeply.

> After Jessica underwent a radical mastectomy for
> breast cancer, she feared that her husband, Jerry, would
> not find her as sexually attractive. When she asked
> him about this issue, he denied that it made any dif-
> ference. Yet he spent longer hours at his office, often
> returning home after Jessica was asleep. She confronted
> him with his behavior. He still insisted that as far as
> he was concerned, her illness had no effect on their
> relationship. Two months after her operation he ad-
> mitted, "I gotta tell you. I can't handle it. I'm leaving."
> Now, a year after their divorce, Jessica says, "Thinking
> back on it, it's probably the best thing to come from
> my cancer."

Expect your relationship with your husband or wife to change in unanticipated ways.

> When their kids finally grew up and moved out,
> Carl and Liz had the chance to do a few "adult"
> things together. They planned to take lessons in social

dancing, for example. But then Carl suddenly got a stroke that paralyzed one side.

After sitting home for the first three months after Carl's stroke, Liz decided to take dance lessons anyway. Carl encouraged her. "It's not something I would have relished before," he explains, "but I hate the idea of Liz having to enter some kind of premature old age just because of me. And when she gets home from those dance classes, she really seems to have a lot more energy for *us*. Under the circumstances, I wouldn't have it any other way."

Don't automatically assume that all changes in the relationship are negative. Some are definitely therapeutic for both of you.

It seemed to Charles that Nelda's arthritis amplified her tendency to complain. He found himself getting angry at her, and finally told her outright. "Other people get arthritis," he said, "and they find more useful things to do than spend the day complaining about it!"

Shocked at first, Nelda realized that Charles was right. This was a feature of her personality she hadn't recognized before and certainly didn't need. "I didn't stop all my complaining," she recalls, "but I stopped most of it, and spent more time doing volunteer work for others. If Charles hadn't blown up at me, I never would have noticed how much time I wasted complaining."

Your spouse needs time off, period. Don't take "no" for an answer.

Mary Ann's friends regarded her as a saint for caring for her husband, Al, as well as she did. Increasingly unable to move because of a neurological disease, Al required more care each week. Mary Ann insisted on doing it all herself, even cleaning up after Al's incontinence.

When she began to curse herself for getting migraine headaches that hampered her work with Al, friends strongly suggested she take time off. Speaking with Al about this, she realized that she had a terrible time relinquishing the sense of control she derived from always being the person on the giving end. Finally friends persuaded her to let them come and care for Al every third evening, giving Mary Ann time to go to films and visit with others. "It was difficult at first," says Mary Ann, "but I feel like a new person now."

Talk about it. When you're finished, talk about it some more.

"I wasn't aware how much Carla's lupus affected our relationship," says Josh. "She usually wasn't outright sick, so we went on about our business. She was more easily fatigued than I'd remembered, so I started to think of her as lazy.

"I guess I started getting angry at her when her sex drive vanished. Then I noticed she was turning down more and more social engagements, supposedly because she couldn't go out in the sun. I began to feel isolated, like I'd been reduced from husband to caretaker.

"I finally blew up at work over some insignificant detail, and my supervisor insisted I go for counseling. That changed my life. I learned to talk — and especially listen — to Carla more honestly than I knew was possible. We're gradually learning that there's nothing that communication can't make better."

Remind each other whom you married. Flesh is known to shift about, being supple at one stage and slack at another. Attractive or repulsive, let's remember that flesh simply ages while less tangible characteristics — generosity, sense of humor, loveableness — endure.

"Dave didn't touch me," confides Sally, "for a year after I got my colostomy. He swore that this change in my appearance was irrelevant, but it was obvious he was repelled." Two months after Sally entered psychotherapy to sort things out, Dave got cancer of the larynx.

"I was amazed Sally still loved me," Dave says through an electronic amplifier. "I thought she'd be disgusted by the loss of my voice, but I learned she really loved me for deeper reasons. And then I realized what a big thing I'd made of her colostomy, and how little it has to do with who she is."

Spend some quiet time together every day. The duration isn't as important as the quality. You don't need to plan a particular event or to even speak. Go for a walk, look at birds together, read to each other, or simply hold hands. Nothing lasts forever.

Richard, a forty-five-year-old artist, developed arm pain and weakness that were diagnosed as severe spinal arthritis. The pain and medication for pain left him unable for weeks to do anything but lay in bed.

"What helped me most during that period," he says, "was when my wife just rested in bed with me and read quietly one hour every day, no matter what. It was like she was telling me, 'Don't worry. Whatever else is happening, I'm here with you.'"

Your Illness and Your Children

For better or worse, families are characteristically well-oiled mechanisms. Never mind whether a family's daily function results in love and support or neurosis and misery. The fact is that families develop unique, usually unrecognized, protocols for their members to deal with one another.

"Tim and I used to spend every minute together, around the clock," Pauline reminisces. "But our first child just required a lot of my time, so Tim and I couldn't be together as much. The second child made even more demands.

"Tim and I hardly saw each other — maybe only in the late evening, when we were tired. That's the way it's been for years, and I guess we've accepted it. When he's home he spends time by himself or with the kids. It's like we barely know each other now. I wonder how it got to be like that."

The complex tapestry of family habits is particularly significant to children. Short on experience and long on dependence, they have few deep connections outside their family. Therefore a change in family dynamics is a relative revolution in the life of a child.

Lacking a history of meaningful comparisons, children are prone to accept whatever is happening as normal. This is not, of course, necessarily bad.

> Jill is a therapist who counsels dying people. Her clients regard her more as a friend than a helping professional, and usually accommodate Jill's request to bring along her eight-year-old, Jessica. Jessica has by now visited the bedsides of dozens of dying people.
>
> "Some of my friends think that's a little weird," says Jessica. "They think dying has something to do with monsters and ghosts. I just tell them it's no big deal."

But if the situation is actually horrid, children will learn a skewed version of what is "normal."

> Nancy wonders about continuing to bring her five-year-old, Mikey, and seven-year-old, Alan, to see their father Ed, who is in the hospital with advanced liver disease. Ed has gotten the notion that his illness is punishment for unspeakable past sins, and he lives his days in mortal fear. If anyone turns off his light at night, he screams until someone turns it on again.
>
> The boys are reluctant to talk about their experiences at the hospital, but Nancy has heard from their teachers that they're both acting out in school and have become problem students. Mikey has begun wetting his bed and insists on sleeping with his light on.

The way children handle chronic illness in the family depends on how the family functions otherwise. A truly communicative family will not likely inflict the twists that require therapy twenty years later. But a family whose currency is vendettas, secrets, taboos, and other neuroses will inevitably decorate the illness with the same old habits. So think of a child's well-being as inextricable from the entire family situation.

Here are a few guideposts for monitoring and influencing your children's reactions to your chronic illness:

Expect the unexpected. Any kind of emotion can surface, even what initially seems inappropriate. Kids might cry, scream, throw temper tantrums, or get gleefully giddy, often with little warning. They are at least as prone as adults to "somatize," to develop physical symptoms and even objective signs like fever and vomiting. Before running them to the emergency room or a social worker, though, gently explore their emotions with them. Surprises are common.

> Jennie and Steve were about to leave for a quiet vacation. A chronic migraine sufferer, Jennie wanted to see if a few days of serenity might obviate the need for medication.
>
> They arranged to leave Martha, their six-year-old daughter, with her favorite aunt. As her parents packed, Martha announced that she didn't feel well and summarily vomited on their bed. Martha had a 104 degree temperature. Steve, a physician, could find no cause for the fever.
>
> They cancelled their vacation plans and spent the next two days working — with little success — to bring Martha's temperature down. Finally a pediatrician friend diagnosed a subtle strep infection and Martha responded rapidly to antibiotics. Says Steve, "It's funny about Martha. As sick as she was, she kept asking if Mom was going to get better. It's as though Martha got sick because she was scared of Jennie leaving." (Jennie and Steve, by the way, finally did enjoy two quiet days together.)

See regression as a sign of stress. Kids generally turn toward the fetal when things look awful to them. They forget their manners, lose vocabulary, wet the bed, and begin to suck their thumbs again. This kind of behavior doesn't mean they've reversed their development, only that they're waving a "Hard Times" sign at you. Assume that regressive behavior is a plea for relief from a stressful situation.

> An exacerbation of Molly's rheumatoid arthritis left her unable to pick up Amy, her five-year-old. Molly, who missed this contact as much as Amy, explained, "Honey, I'd love to pick you up. It just hurts my back too much."
>
> Over the next few days, Amy complained diffusely of problems with walking. One morning she gravely announced, "Momma, I can't walk at all today. Now you have to carry me." Molly cried most of the morning but spent the afternoon lying in bed with Amy, reading to her. By evening Amy was walking, bringing her mother food and juice.

Seek outside help for your child if an emotion or unhealthy behavior becomes chronic. Denial, anger, fear, regression, disorientation, and all the other responses that can occur are either finite or tractable in everyone, child or adult, if confronted appropriately. If a child remains, say, fearful day after day despite the best interventions of other family members, seek professional help. This is especially true for depression.

> Simone, a thirty-eight-year-old single mother with asthma, was managing with herculean effort to raise her nine-year-old daughter and hold a responsible job with a bank. Whenever she had an asthmatic attack she wondered whether it had been brought on by the stress of trying to do too much. "More than once," she says, "I thought to myself, 'Do I have to choose between working and raising Sadie?'"
>
> Simone began to notice that Sadie was gaining weight. She learned that Sadie had been eating compulsively for months, sneaking huge amounts of candy between meals. She talked with Sadie about this, but all she discovered, unsurprisingly, was that Sadie wished her mom was home more. When she wasn't working, Simone spent significantly more time with her

daughter. "But it didn't help much," says Simone. "Sadie kept gaining weight and I got asthma attacks more often."

When Simone finally consulted a therapist, she learned that her most important value was "...to support my daughter." She came to see that the support she needed to give was direct support, at home, rather than the financial support she had almost exclusively focused on. She also came to see Sadie's overeating as a symbolic message that although her material needs were more than met, she hungered for nourishment nonetheless. Simone arranged to take several months off her job. Living on their savings, she and Sadie had a great time with each other and Sadie's weight returned to normal.

Reread the suggestions I made for what you and your spouse can do to protect your relationship. They are equally applicable to you and your kids. Since chronic illness invariably shuffles the family deck, why not shuffle toward healthier communication?

Your Illness and Your Friends

Again, no one gets off the hook. Everyone's affected one way or another by your illness. Old family friends, fishing buddies, card partners, and office mates will, without exception, have their own particular reaction. Whether they express it overtly or not, they are sure to enact it.

Friends can get disoriented. For example, perhaps they've been used to dealing with you as Good Time Rita or Joe the Joker, and now you're apparently someone else. How should they relate?

Friends can be fearful. Frankly, your illness can scare the bejabbers out of them. Maybe they think it's contagious or maybe it unconsciously revives a past they've repressed. Maybe they'd just as soon not face their own depression. Maybe some calculator inside them figures you won't be around for the office party. Maybe an unspoken farewell is their implicit acknowledgment of your illness. So you discover that a few old buddies won't look you in the eye or don't even come around anymore, and the folks at the office forget to invite you to the annual picnic.

It's important to remind yourself in sad situations like these that other people's actions are based on their own belief systems, not necessarily on what's actually happening with you.

Most of all, though, your friends love you. They can't easily bear to see you in pain or contemplate your demise. They will offer you the latest in diets for your condition. They'll phone with addresses of avant-garde clinics. They'll talk your ear off about Great-Aunt Tessie's watermelon seed cure and Grandpa Futz' mustard poultice. They'll loan you walls of books, bushels of instructive audiotapes. The space around your bed will begin to resemble a library after an earthquake. Your friends want you cured, and now.

It's hardest to be a good friend when your friend is sick. The most common question I hear from friends of sick people is, "But what do I say?" After all, they want to give you support, hope, and cheer. The answer is the same as if no one were sick: you don't need to say anything. Sometimes the best healing tools are a finely tuned ear and an open heart.

> "I noticed that when my friends visited me in the hospital after my cancer operation," says Dorothy, "they tended to do one of two things. Some of them told me what I'd need to do to get better and others just asked me how I was doing. And they meant it. They actually wanted to hear what it was that I was going through.
>
> "Now, that made me think. Sometimes I didn't even know my feelings until I began to speak. Sometimes I was surprised by what I said. In fact, now that I'm out of the hospital I just want to keep acting like that. I've never learned so much about myself in my whole life! It's too bad that it took cancer to bring this about, but if that's what was needed, well...I know that's a strange thing to say, isn't it?"

Knowing that your friends want the best for you in their own unique ways, here are a few suggestions to bring out the best:

Make your changes easy on your friends. When they seem distraught and helpless, recall that *they share your illness* — so simply ask them how it is for them. I guarantee a fruitful conversation will ensue.

> "When I was fishing with Paul, my arthritis kept me from opening the bait jar," recalls Gene. "I couldn't unscrew the thing no matter how hard I tried, and it hurt like hell. I looked up and saw Paul watching me.
> "He was wringing his hands and had the most God-awful look on his face, as if he was watching his mother get run over. I said, 'Paul, it looks to me like you're having more trouble with this damn jar than I am.' Well, he laughed so hard he almost cried, and then we talked for awhile about my arthritis."

Accept with sincere gratitude whatever kind of help friends offer, even though you may believe it to be useless or even harmful. As with any gift, the substance is less important than the intent.

Recognize and enforce priorities. One side benefit of chronic and serious illness is the sense of vulnerability and mortality that may not have been there before: time becomes more valuable. Guard your time. Choose which friends you will see and for how long. Gently decline to be with those people whom you've always seen exclusively out of politeness. After all, your illness is a perfectly acceptable generic excuse, isn't it?

Ask for help. Since they usually can't do much about your disease, friends can feel helpless. Ease their frustration by asking for something they can provide. I feel good when I say I love you, and even better when I show it.

Exercise: Assertiveness

When your normal capabilities are compromised by sickness, you'll find it useful to state your needs as clearly as possible. You needn't scream your needs or whine them, but simply state them.

That is, aggression and passivity will not usually serve you as well as assertiveness. Here are some examples of different communication styles:

> *Aggressive:* "It's hot in here, damnit! How come I'm always the one who has to notice it first? You all think that just because I can't move around, you can forget about me."

> *Passive:* "Is the temperature in here okay for you? I'm not sure, because one of my medicines wrecks my sense of temperature; but it kind of seems a little bit too warm. Do you think it's too warm?"

> *Assertive:* "It's pretty warm in here. In fact, I'm uncomfortable. I'd appreciate it if you'd turn the heat down."

An aggressive statement can be loud, angry, and callous; a passive statement can be weak and hedging; an assertive statement is honest and direct. Although aggression and passivity are occasionally appropriate, it's the assertive style that will most often get you what you need without undue agony.

Notice that my assertive statement has three parts:

1. My view of the situation: "It's pretty warm in here."
2. My feelings about the situation: "I'm uncomfortable."
3. My wants: "…turn the heat down."

Think carefully about a real personal need, and about the person with whom you'd have to speak to have that need fulfilled. In your illness journal, write exactly what you would say to this person, but in all three styles: aggressive, passive, and assertive. Exaggerate the styles and have fun with them. Which style do you tend to use most often? Have you noticed your communication style more since you've been ill? Remember when writing your assertive statement to include your view of the situation, your feelings about it, and your wants.

Review what you've written, noting the wide expressive range available to you. Finally, go to the person who can satisfy your need, and actually express yourself assertively. Record the physical result of this transaction, along with your emotional experience.

Exercise: Getting Centered

With diligent practice, you can voluntarily maximize your serenity within most situations. This is a method I use to teach emergency room personnel — who frequently find themselves immersed in a half-dozen simultaneous crises — to stay "centered." My mentor in this area is Rudyard Kipling, who offered this ideal: "If you can keep your head when all about you are losing theirs and blaming it on you..."

Read and understand the complete instructions before you begin so that you will not need to interrupt yourself.

1. As usual, assure yourself of ten minutes of quiet solitude. Request that your family not approach you or speak with you *after* this exercise until you speak to them.

2. Lie on your back comfortably, getting the sense that you're using so little energy you're falling into the bed. Close your eyes but do not drift off or sleep. If you do fall asleep, take heart and try again tomorrow.

3. As in previous exercises, place your attention fully in your breath. When mental chatter intervenes — and it will — gently and persistently return your attention exclusively to the breath. Again, don't be tough on yourself: honor the fact that chatter is tenacious.

4. After some practice you will note that at least for a few seconds at a time you are chatter-free, breathing without thinking. Congratulations! The next step is to test your skill a bit by opening your eyes. Let them blink and roll around as they will, but keep them softly passive, as though they are seeing without looking.

5. When you feel confident with this, sit up. Notice that opening the eyes and initiating any movement increases the challenge to your concentration. If your attention leaves your breath as you arise, lie down and try again.

6. Test your skill further by standing. If you can still maintain a silent mind, walk. Walk slowly around your room simply for the experience of ambulating without thinking. You are centered now,

inhabiting the real world without being yanked about by your usual emotional hooks. Feels strange, doesn't it? But as you experience this, deliberately feel it throughout your body in whatever intensity you can manage. Don't conjure words about it. Your body will memorize the experience simply by feeling it. And once it's there you won't forget it.

7. When you feel comfortable with the previous step, open the door and circulate through the house among other family members. You've already asked them not to approach or speak with you, so you needn't worry about interruption. Consider this: here you are, walking around in your home among your family and still totally serene. Sense as fully as you can what this condition feels like.

8. End the exercise by talking with your family. Describe to them what the exercise felt like. Guide them in it if they wish to try it themselves. Recall this centered feeling at will, renovating it occasionally with practice. As you become more confident with this skill, try it out within progressively more stressful situations — such as when an unwanted caller drops by, or the person in line in front of you at the grocery store begins a lengthy argument with the clerk. You may eventually come to see a centered, quiet mind as the normal state of being.

5

Your Illness
and Your Doctor

Choosing a Doctor

Your choice of doctor is crucial. All else equal, the relationship between you and your doctor can be as therapeutic as medical treatment.

> Eight-year-old Anthony saw Dr. Parker, a family physician, because of warts on Anthony's hands. Dr. Parker said, "These are little infections, Anthony. They probably won't spread or get larger. There are two ways I can treat them. I can burn them off with a chemical or you can go home and wish them away. Now, which would you like to do?" "I can wish them away?" asked Anthony. "Of course you can. Kids do it all the time." Anthony went home, wished, and his warts were gone within two weeks.
>
> * * *
>
> After reviewing breast cancer statistics with Elena, her surgeon asked her to go home and decide between a lumpectomy — limited local excision — and a mastec-

tomy. She phoned her family physician, Dr. Wilson, and asked his opinion.

"Well, Elena," he said, "I've known you fifteen years. How would you characterize yourself? Would you say you're fairly compulsive?"

"Compulsive?" she responded. "Are you talking about my insistence on covering details? You bet!"

"Exactly. With that in mind, might you worry about whether a lumpectomy missed a few cancer cells?"

"I hadn't thought about it like that, but I guess I would. When I do something, I like to finish it totally so that I don't have to think about it anymore."

"Does that knowledge about yourself suggest a choice to you?"

Elena thought about it one more day and chose the mastectomy. "I'm so glad I had Dr. Wilson to ask," she says. "He knows medicine and he also knows who I am."

If this were a book about disease — the physical manifestation of sickness — I'd simply direct you to the physician best qualified to treat disease. I'd recommend that you make sure the doctor is recognized as an expert in his or her specialty, or what's called in medicine "board-certified." I'd recommend that you learn if he or she has a teaching position in a medical training institution. I'd recommend that you ask other doctors how often they ask the doctor in question to consult on their own patients.

But this is a book about illness — your personal experience — so the requirements are more comprehensive. You're looking for a doctor with technical *and human* qualities, someone who can approach your disease as disordered physiology and at the same time recognize and seek to alleviate your suffering. This breadth, as a matter of fact, distinguishes an authentic healer from a merely competent technician. When you find such people, treasure them.

Dr. Louis Behm was Chief of Medicine at a prestigious teaching hospital. His students said he knew everything about medicine. But he also exhibited unusual calm and humility. Every Thursday at noon he conducted grand rounds in the hospital's large auditorium. Hundreds of residents, interns, and medical students attended.

The patient of the week was wheeled in. This was a very sick person, extensively jaundiced, thin, and withdrawn. His internal medicine resident presented the case — the history, physical examination, test results, diagnosis, treatment, and course.

Most members of the audience followed the resident's presentation, but a few eyes wandered to Dr. Behm, who stood quietly behind the patient, bent over him, sat beside him. Dr. Behm continually touched the man: when he wasn't palpating his abdomen, Dr. Behm was massaging his shoulders.

Then Dr. Behm delivered a lecture about the disease in an organized style that came from decades of deep experience. In all this he continued to touch the sick man, who now paid as diligent attention to the lecture as did anyone in the room.

Finally questions were asked and answered and the patient, by now more pink than yellow, was returned to the ward.

Here are a few simple suggestions for initiating a quest for your own healing relationship.

Check out the doctor's professional credentials. Make a list of doctors in your area who practice the specialty you need. Verify their medical credentials, because even Dr. Humane can amputate the wrong leg. You can do this simply by phoning your county medical association or State Board of Medical Quality Assurance.

Question the doctor's patients. Ask friends and relatives for the names of people who have been seen by the doctors on your list. Phone these patients. They'll probably be happy to discuss their doctor with you. Ask questions such as these, amending them to your preferences:

- Can you reach the doctor easily by phone?

- Is there much of a wait in the waiting room?

- When there is a wait, does the doctor express concern about your time?

- Is the staff friendly and courteous, and do they place you before their paperwork?

- Do you have access to your medical records?

- Is the doctor on an equivalent-name basis with you (i.e., Dr./Ms. or Harry/Sarah), or does the doctor use your first name while retaining the title "Doctor"?

- Is the doctor comfortable with emotion?

- Does the doctor meet you — when you're fully clothed — in an office setting before or after examinations, or are conversations confined to the examining room, where you're wearing a paper gown?

- Does the doctor warm instruments (stethoscope, vaginal speculum) before touching you with them?

- Does the doctor express concern for your suffering?

- Does the doctor ask you what you feel your problem is, and then respect your appraisal?

- Does the doctor reveal enough about his/her life to make you feel that you have a personal relationship?

- Does the doctor touch you caringly? Pat or hug you?

Don't take one person's story as total gospel, for everyone has a particular tilt. So try to reach at least two patients of each physician, and consider trends to be more significant than specific answers. The information you gather from these people will narrow your list.

Interview the remaining prospects. Phone the doctor in question, offering to pay his or her rate for a fifteen-minute interview. *This is time and money well-spent.* For one thing, without any cost you'll immediately weed out those who don't think enough of your individual needs to grant a paid interview.

Consider the interview as a blind date. In a way it is, since it may be the first meeting in an important — and possibly lifelong — relationship. Just as I wouldn't presume to dictate your conversation on a date, I won't do so here.

No matter what you and the doctor speak about in this brief conversation, you'll learn volumes about your ability to form a powerful partnership with this person. Note the doctor's relative warmth, apparent personal health and stress level, physical and eye contact, concern, sense of humor, and even the furniture arrangement (e.g., do you want a desk between the two of you? Are there works of art on the walls, or an inspiring view?).

From these interviews you ought to be able to compose a preference list of physicians. You may even be drawn to more than one of the doctors.

"I figured it was *my* body," says Ida, "so I wouldn't go to just anybody. I used to go to Dr. Wald, but she always struck me as a cold fish. I wanted someone more personable. Anyway, I thought I'd give her another chance, so I called her and said I wanted to see her again, but just to talk. She said fine, come talk.

"In her office I told her I wanted to know her ideas about treating people like me. Not her medical ideas, but her ideas about people. Well, did she come alive! It was like instant person. She told me she went into medicine to work with people, and that she'd been disappointed during her whole career because it seemed like her patients just wanted an engineer. She said my visit gave her new hope. Well, anyway, it made my day. So she's still my doctor and we're doing fine."

What To Expect From Your Doctor

Once established, the healing relationship should be deep and intimate. The analogy of a marriage is apt again, for this partnership requires ongoing fine-tuning. You will both need constantly to assert your needs and determine your responsibilities.

Besides the requirement of technical competence, there is only one thing you should continually expect from your doctor: *expect and demand a healing relationship.*

This means that your doctor relates to you before relating to your disease. You — as you are in the instant of your visit — are more important than your chart, your test results, or your blood pressure. Your needs, fears, anxieties, and strengths are as real and operant as your disease, and need at least the same careful appreciation given to any blood test or body part.

As you're probably aware, we medical doctors are fascinated by technology. It's unfortunate, but our training tends to leave us more comfortable with machinery than with people. So it is that we tend to feel shaky with patients until we can pull a frame of words and numbers around them. This predisposition damages our own humanity and limits our ability to heal as much as it degrades our patients; so for your sake and ours, please keep reminding us how important you are.

What To Expect From Yourself

You've chosen your doctor at least partly for his or her partnership skills, which means you're necessarily an active partner as well. Here are some ways you can participate:

Above all, communicate your feelings and needs. The first time I was struck by the necessity for this advice was when I asked a new patient, "What seems to be the problem?" and he replied, "You tell me. You're the doctor."

Doctors aren't trained clairvoyants. It's up to you to say what's on your mind. This isn't always easy. Many patients get disoriented and intimidated simply by being in a medical office; the statements and questions they carefully formulated at home evaporate into thin air. Or they might believe that the doctor is too busy to wade through all their questions, or that their concerns are trivial. But if you've followed the game plan in this book, you've selected a doctor who is interested in you and who does have time for you.

So make it easy for both of you by getting more actively involved. Do your homework: before your appointment, think carefully about what you want to say and ask. Write your concerns, leaving room on the paper to write responses during your visit. If you seem to have forgotten your doctor's comments during the previous visit, bring a portable tape recorder next time. If neces-

sary, bring a friend — especially if you anticipate that significantly emotional issues will arise.

**Inform your doctor that you'll want to know the rationale
for every test he or she orders.** This keeps doctors on their in-
tellectual toes. More often than you may think, doctors order
"routine" tests whether they're really needed or not. Sometimes
they order tests not for diagnostic reasons, but to avoid potential
liability or for academic interest. Since every test inevitably involves some combination of time, expense, pain, and/or hazard,
ask your doctor, *"How will a given result from this test change what
you do?"*

> At the age of eighty-eight, Murray isn't in bad shape.
> But his doctor diagnosed Murray's dizzy spell two
> weeks ago as a "transient ischemic attack."
> "That means, Murray," the doctor explained, "that
> your brain might not be getting all the blood it needs.
> I suspect there are obstructions in one of the arteries in
> your neck that go to your brain." The doctor told Mur-
> ray that he'd like to do a carotid arteriogram, in which
> x-ray-sensitive dye would be injected into Murray's
> arteries to reveal blockage.
> "Why do the test?" asked Murray.
> "Well, so we'll know what's wrong, of course."
> "I repeat," said Murray, "Why do the test? What
> will you do with the results?"
> "It depends on what the test shows."
> "C'mon, doc. Are you going to operate on me?
> Are the risks worth it in an eighty-eight-year-old man?"
> "Murray, your brain is in better shape than mine."

Ask about all your treatment options. There are always
choices. Keep in mind that one option in any situation is to do
nothing.

Ask your doctor if she would choose for herself what she
recommends. I've found doctors generally candid when asked
this question. Studies, by the way, show that members of doctors'
families often opt for treatments outside "mainstream" medicine.

The choice in every case must ultimately be up to you. If
you choose a course that differs from your doctor's recommen-

dation, recruit her cheerful assent. A doctor who begrudges your choice, no matter how foolish it seems to her, is not respecting your personhood; you'll need to have an attitudinal adjustment session together.

> Cora suffered from a large neck tumor for which she'd been treated repeatedly. Now her surgeon told her it could be removed only with a major operation that would leave her markedly disfigured, and that the tumor would probably return anyway.
> A timid lady in her seventies, Cora spoke her feelings about the proposed operation at her cancer support group. "I just don't want any more surgery," she said, "but I've never gone against my doctor's wishes."
> "Cora," suggested a group member, "why don't you just say no anyway?"
> "Oh, my! Say no? Just say no?" Cora was clearly both frightened and titillated by the prospect.
> The next week another group member asked why Cora looked so "up."
> "Well," Cora said, "I saw my surgeon and I told her, 'I don't believe I'll have that operation, and the surgeon told me, 'You know what? I don't think I'd have that operation, either!'"

Request access to your medical records. Not too long ago, prescriptions were written in Latin and nurses weren't allowed even to tell you your blood pressure. It was felt that patients did best when all knowledge was left in the doctor's hands.

Times have changed. With some additional training, nurses can now practice essentially as doctors in many states. Any number of drugs available only by prescription yesterday are sold over-the-counter today. And more patients have access to their medical records.

Ask your doctor for access to your records. The right to browse and copy your records means that nothing of substance is being kept from you. Your doctor knows that there can be no secrets about diagnosis, for example, or what consultants have written. Access means that you can bring the records to someone else to interpret for you. It means that any other practitioner you visit will have the benefit of seeing an organized medical history.

Balance faith in your doctor with knowledge of his falli-bility. Go into every treatment accepting that it can possibly entail adverse consequences *and* that your doctor's doing his best. Ask about the potential hazards involved in specific treatments and in declining those treatments.

The best way to wreck a healing relationship is to proceed with unspoken skepticism and then suffer injury. Impressive statistics reveal that the majority of medical liability ("malpractice") suits come not necessarily from actual malpractice, but from a faulty relationship.

> Mona weighed almost 400 pounds last year. "I've never stuck to a diet more than a few hours," she says. "I guess I've got an addictive personality. I found out about Dr. Collins through friends. He does this operation where he removes so much of your intestine that you can't digest much anymore. And while he's in there he cuts out a lot of belly fat, too. Sounded like what I wanted, so I went to him. Actually, I spent more time with his nurse than with him. He just felt my belly and set a date. Told me he's never had any trouble with the operation, so I believed him.
>
> "I still believe him. *He's* never had any trouble with the operation, but I've had plenty. I've lost over two hundred pounds, but I spend most of my day in the bathroom. Whatever I put in one end falls out the other. I complained to Dr. Collins, but he said the operation went perfectly and that he'd told me this would happen afterward. Well, I'm suing him for malpractice. Doctors shouldn't be allowed to do that kind of thing to people."

When this happens, both parties are characteristically at fault. The patient tosses a ridiculously unhealthy chunk of responsibility into the doctor's lap and the doctor is ego-driven enough to accept it. Any relationship this lopsided is obviously begging for trouble.

In weighing the potential treatment hazards your doctor describes for you, remember that you may not fit handily into the statistics. Take into account how your life deviates from the theoretical average. You may, for example, be in better shape than most people who face similar surgery. You may have a consistent history of slower healing. Or you know you'll be able to leave the hospital earlier than other patients because you have abundant support at home.

Tell your doctor about any new symptoms. Don't assume that new symptoms are an extension of your disease, for they will often be side effects or toxic effects of treatment, and may be remediable.

"I was worried sick," says Madge. "Dr. Bonney gave me these pills for my arthritis. He told me I might get a little stomach discomfort from them, but he didn't tell me I'd double over in pain. I was getting the same kind of pains as my friend Linda did when she got stomach cancer. I thought, 'My God, arthritis isn't enough! I've probably got stomach cancer, too!' I was so frightened, I avoided calling Dr. Bonney for a week. But then it got so bad I had to call him. He just took me off those pills and the pain disappeared."

Insist upon your dignity. I perennially suggest that health professionals experience patienthood. One reason is for them to see how degrading the experience can be. Without even being aware of it, medical (and, yes, "alternative") institutions and the people who compose them can be uncaring, intrusive, condescending, coarse, presumptuous, insolent, and even brutal. I've seen such behavior commonly in hospitals, and, in a more ignorant phase, have been guilty of some myself.

I don't raise this issue in regard to your regular doctor, since I assume you are steadily refining that relationship. But you can't always choose the people who work with you. You will probably come into contact with consulting physicians, technicians, students, physical therapists, nurses, and maintenance and housekeeping staff with whom you have no prior relationship and therefore neither familiarity nor a mutual agreement for behavior.

There are reasons why people who enter this nominally delicate, genial calling might act so contrary. Most often it's because they're frightened of sickness and consequently frightened of those who manifest it. Perhaps they are overworked, underpaid, and underappreciated. Perhaps they react to the constant tragedy around them by steeling their souls. And occasionally this unconscious insensitivity becomes institutionalized, a behavioral norm. Whatever the cause and extent, though, it's intolerable, both for you and, of course, for them.

If practitioners treat you this way, the only effective response you can offer is to insist on your dignity. To blow up at them will not change things; it will probably only make your day worse. Besides, they are doing their best within their current personal limitations, so forgive them and continue to insist on your dignity until they realize they simply must change their approach.

John Marshall, a seventy-five-year-old man, lived in his own room in a board-and-care home. He fell one night, breaking his hip. Though elderly, he was thought strong enough to undergo a corrective operation. He came through it successfully and was sent to a convalescent hospital to recuperate.

On his third day in this hospital, a young man in a white smock came to his bed and loudly announced, "Time for your physical therapy, John!" The man and his assistant moved John to a wheelchair. John cried in pain. "We know it hurts, John," the young man shouted, "but you need PT so you can heal." The man wheeled John to the physical therapy room, where he tried to get him to stand with a walker. "C'mon, big guy!" he shouted in encouragement.

John thought this fellow might indeed do him good, but something about his manner grated him. It crystallized when the young man loudly exclaimed, "Attaboy! Attaboy! You're gonna be back on your feet in no time and wowing the girls back home, aren't you, John?"

John mustered all his strength to lock his elbows so that he could remain standing with the walker. "Young man," he began, "I don't know who you are. You didn't introduce yourself. But I will. I am Mr. Marshall. Please don't call me 'John.' And I'm not deaf, so you don't have to shout. I am a human being, and I expect to be treated like one. Please send for your supervisor and go find someone else to work with until you can show some respect for me."

The supervisor was surprised by John's criticism. "But no one's complained before," he said.

"That doesn't matter," said John. "No one's ever treated me like a nonentity, and while I have a say about it, no one will."

"But the therapist was just being friendly," explained the supervisor.

John looked the man in the eye. "I believe you heard what I told you," he said. "Now please give it due consideration."

After that moment, John received nothing but courteous attention. His roommate confided to John the next day, "Hey, have you noticed that they've stopped shouting?"

Choosing a Nondoctor

Not everyone chooses a practitioner of standard medicine. Nonphysicians are seen by more people today than at any time in the past generation. They get diagnosed and treated by chiropractors, massage and bodywork practitioners, acupuncturists, nutritionists, faith healers, and many others. It's not uncommon for patients to see a few practitioners — including a medical doctor — concurrently.

If you're interested in finding a nonmedical practitioner, look beyond such verbal descriptions as "holistic." Holistic is in the same category of adjectives as "new," "improved," and "organic." The problem is that words and the realities they represent can be shockingly disparate. I've never met a medical doctor who didn't claim to treat "the whole patient." If we're not all holistic, at least we say we are. Conversely, I've known "alternative" practitioners who are more coldly mechanistic than the most impersonal physician you'd care to name.

The problem is that none of us can comprehend a more "whole" person than we recognize in ourselves. People with narrow vision who claim to enjoy a whole view lack more in insight than sincerity. Their work as healers is cut out for them, for the words "heal" and "whole" share a common root. The ancient admonition "Healer, heal thyself" has as much relevance today as ever.

Doug and Mitch are the partners in a cardiology practice. Putting it mildly, they are both highly strung individuals. Their eyes pop and veins bulge with the slightest effort. Some of their patients joke that their office smells like an adrenaline distillery, and even worry about these doctors having premature heart attacks.

But from the doctors' vantage point, things don't look so pessimistic. Every year Doug and Mitch trade physical exams, and every year each gives the other a clean bill of health.

It's not for me to encourage you to see either medical or "alternative" practitioners or a combination. This is exclusively your option. But I do encourage you as strongly as I can to *choose an approach and practitioner most congruent with your beliefs*. Continual review of your illness journal should furnish substantial clues as to what these beliefs are.

If you suspect, in your heart of hearts, that kissing light bulbs will cure you, then indeed it may. Someone, somewhere, will testify enthusiastically to almost any approach. On the other hand, doubts about a treatment will likely reduce your compliance with and response to that treatment. For example, if you regard cancer chemotherapy as harsh and poisonous, I'd expect a dismal outcome. In my mind, one of modern medicine's most poignant failings is the dismissal of the power of patients' belief systems, or what we call the "placebo effect."

Violeta, a thirty-three-year-old Filipina, developed what her doctor diagnosed as a gallstone. He recommended surgery. She said, "I told him that since I was about to visit relatives in Manila, I'd see a friend of the family who's a psychic surgeon. My doctor didn't like that at all."

Upon arriving in the Philippines, Violeta fasted and prayed for a week, then saw the psychic surgeon. After massaging her belly, he seemed to extract bloody material from it without incising her skin. "I don't know exactly what he did," said Violeta. "Maybe it's magic, maybe it's a trick. But when I came home and got new X-rays, my doctor told me that the stone was gone."

* * *

Ray, a thirty-five-year-old avid tennis player, developed chronic left knee pain. His orthopedist, Dr. Genasci, told him he'd badly injured the cartilage within the joint, and that a rather simple operation would probably provide him permanent relief.

"But I'd never had surgery," said Ray. "I'd never needed it, and didn't think I needed it then. I figured that what the knee needed was a rest."

Ray, however, couldn't rest. "I played in a tournament almost every weekend. One Sunday I had to be carried off the court."

He visited Dr. Genasci again. The doctor asked, "What is it that you have against surgery?" In the ensuing dialog, Ray realized his principal objection was to general anesthesia. "I couldn't stand being totally at someone else's mercy. I don't know why. It just bothered me a lot."

After conferring with an anesthesiologist, Dr. Genasci offered Ray spinal anesthesia, in which he would be fully conscious. Ray finally opted for this, underwent the surgery, and healed perfectly. He continues to play in tournaments.

There's another reason I ask you to choose an approach most consistent with your belief system. Your friends and relatives will probably feed you more information about practices and practitioners than you can digest in a sitting, and you may experience a desire to follow virtually every lead. Some people, driven by desperation, rush through clinics from Sonora to Singapore. They adopt radically different diets monthly. They submit themselves as often as possible to treatments that can be drastic, hazardous, exhausting, mutually conflicting, and as ludicrous as they are expensive.

The seductive kicker, of course, is that a few of these people show demonstrable cures.

Even so, I oppose this strategy because it skims the surface of possibilities at the cost of depth. It limits your ability to learn from your sickness. It fills what could be valuable creative time with a disease obsession. Economics aside, it is too expensive spiritually.

> Millie, sixty years old, is angry and frustrated. The past five years she's lived on the remnants of her late husband's life insurance. When she developed lung cancer last year she looked for nonmedical cures.
> "I wasn't interested in chemotherapy," she said. "I went to Mexico and received Laetrile, along with a strict diet and coffee enemas. Someone there told me about a clinic in Hungary that treated cancer with certain enzymes, so I went for that, too. But that used up almost all my money, so when I heard about a wonderful new treatment in the Bahamas, I couldn't afford to go. I'm furious about this. I've been writing to my congressman. I'm sure that the Bahamas treatment would cure me, but I can't get the money to get into the program."

If a nonmedical approach interests you, subject its practitioners to the same technical and personal scrutiny you would apply to a medical doctor.

Guidelines for Making a Choice

You'll need to investigate nonmedical practitioners a little differently than you would medical doctors. Some degree of skepticism is in order, for when the call went out for a thousand flowers to bloom, many weeds appeared.

In addition, most "alternative" practices haven't enjoyed a popularity comparable to that of standard medicine. Therefore they aren't as organized or as standardized, and this is both good — in its latitude for experimentation — and bad — in that it will be harder for you to verify the *significance* of the credentials of both the practice and practitioner. For example, is a Palmer chiropractic graduate more competent than one who took a different route? Is Rolfing more beneficial than Alexander body work? When you see the letters "L.Ac." after your acupuncturist's name, what can you surmise about his or her competence?

Here are some pointers for your quest:

Match a prospective healing discipline with your beliefs.
Becoming familiar with elements of your own belief system,
you'll more likely select an approach that's congruent with it.

If you believe your sickness to be a matter of disordered
physiology, you'll probably do best with a medical doctor. If you
see it as disharmony with natural powers, you may want to consult a Native American shaman or a drugless practitioner.
Chinese doctors see sickness as an imbalance of the *yin* and *yang*
forces that flow through the body. Chiropractors understand disease principally as a disruption of precise vertebral alignment. To
many body workers, a sickness expresses messages about the person's lifelong habits. This list could continue for several pages. If
you have mixed ideas about your sickness, consider a combination of practitioners.

> Maureen has long been bothered by Raynaud's
> phenomenon, a sudden loss of blood supply to the
> fingers thought to be caused by an underlying, occult
> disease.
> "I must have gone to six or seven doctors to try to
> learn what was causing it," she says. "I thought the
> problem was the difficulty of diagnosis. Then I saw Dr.
> Talbot and discovered the problem was that the other
> doctors hadn't included God in the solution. Like me,
> Dr. Talbot is a committed Christian. He and I pray
> together whenever I visit him. He seeks God's
> guidance in finding my treatment, and I'm sure he'll
> get it."

Learn what's available. A complete review of the nature of
all alternative practices is outside the scope of this book. Details
about these practices are available elsewhere; I've listed a couple
of sources in the "Further Reading" section.

To learn the range of practitioners in your community, begin by consulting the yellow pages of your telephone book. My
local book — and I live in a rural county of only 80,000 people —
lists acupuncturists, biofeedback practitioners, chiropractors,
counselors, disabled services, drugless and holistic practitioners,
homeopaths, hypnotists, massage practitioners, nutritionists,
physicians, psychologists, and yoga instructors. And the phone

book is only one source. Some of the finest healers don't advertise. As a matter of fact, a few aren't even aware that they're healers.

At seventeen, Vicki has been treated for facial acne for five years. "I've tried it all," she says. "Wash your face every ten minutes, no pizzas, no chocolate, keep out of the sun, get more sun, whatever. I just got tired of it. I'd really like to have a social life. All my friends have been dating for years, but who'd want to date me? So I started asking people what to do about it besides xeroxed diets and stupid restrictions.

"I asked a lot of kids, even boys. I asked Eli, who's an incredible nerd. He said he cleared his up by going to all the horror movies he could find. I told him that sounded dumb, but I figured, 'What can I lose?' I went to *The Night of the Living Dead* with Eli, and halfway through I realized this was like a date. Then I thought, 'No, it's a treatment.' Well, whatever it was, Eli was right. He and I have gone to a different horror movie every weekend for two months now, and my face has just about cleared up."

In researching a practice, don't ask people who have an interest in the issue. A friend of mind invariably asks servers in restaurants, "Is the food good here?" They've never said no, and he still hasn't caught on that people tend to favor their own wares over others'. So don't spin your wheels by doing what my friend does. I wouldn't, for example, ask either a chiropractor or a medical doctor about chiropractic — both will have a prejudiced point of view.

How old is the practice? Determine how the discipline has withstood the test of time. Has it endured for centuries or even millenia, like yoga, herbal therapy, surgery, and acupuncture, or was it invented a couple of years ago?

Ask for a reading list. Does the discipline seem to be regarded highly by people outside its own circle, or is its entire literature composed of passionate tracts written by its practitioners? Do practitioners publish journals in which they debate theory, evaluate treatments, and in general communicate with one another?

Ask about the practitioner's training. In particular, ask his or her training *lineage*: "Who trained you? Who trained your teacher? Who trained your teacher's teacher?" Look for knowledge passed from the core of a discipline rather than from its periphery. In medical terms, I'd feel more comfortable with a doctor whose educational "grandfather" was a towering figure such as Sir William Osler than someone I'd never heard of.

In addition, ask about ongoing training. How does the practitioner stay current with new developments in the field?

Speak with patients. Any practitioner worth his or her salt will either give you people's names or ask them to contact you. Ask them the same questions you would ask about a medical doctor. As usual, evaluate their stories judiciously.

Figure practice economics. Estimate wages and other costs in the practice to see whether they jibe with what you are being charged. I've occasionally seen what can only be described as a scandalously gross disparity that indicates more of a money mill than a *bona fide* healing center.

Interview the practitioner. All else equal, you're looking for a partner in what may be a long-term relationship. Interview your prospects in the same way you'd interview a medical doctor.

Above all, use common sense. That is, trust the evidence of your own senses. Demand demystification. Ask the practitioner to explain the nature of your disorder and its proposed treatment. If the practitioner can't or won't explain it to your satisfaction, it's not for you. This is as true for medical doctors as it is for other practitioners.

Ward and Myrna learned about Dr. B., a medical doctor who treated prostate cancer with intravenous chemicals instead of standard medications or surgery. "Let's check him out, Myrna," said Ward. "Maybe I can get his medicines instead of an operation."

They were shown around the clinic by Dr. B. himself. In the treatment room, where a dozen patients received their intravenous treatments on soft recliners drawn into a circle, Myrna asked, "How does your treatment work, Dr. B.?" "Oh," he replied, "a combination of chelation and megadosage," and moved on to the laboratory.

On the ride home Ward said, "That was impressive. An awful lot of people believe in Dr. B." Myrna replied, "Ward, I think he's a phony." They continued their discussion into the night, finally deciding not to embark upon any treatment they both didn't fully accept.

Exercise: Choosing a Doctor

Let's suppose you've narrowed your list of possible practitioners to the three or four you've interviewed. How will you determine your preference? In this exercise you'll fine-tune your needs and match them to what the practitioner offers.

1. List five qualities you demand from a practitioner, and rate them in the order of importance to you on a scale from 1 to 5, with 1 being the most important and 5 being the least important.

Tom, who's looking for relief from chronic back pain, made his list of qualities and ranked them in importance:

	Priority
Interest in me	2
Demonstrated competence in the discipline	1
Reasonable fees	5
Sense of humor	4
Easy access, since I can't easily climb stairs	3

2. In your illness journal, construct a chart that lists the qualities — in your ranked order — in the left column, and then a column for each practitioner. Here's Tom's chart:

Qualities	Dr. Wilson, orthopedics	Dr. Chan, acupuncture	Mary Smith, physical therapy
1. Competence			
2. Interest			
3. Access			
4. Humor			
5. Fees			

3. Now rate each practitioner in each category, assigning more possible points to the more important qualities. Use the following weighted scale (1 is lowest, 10 is highest):

Quality 1: 1-10 points
Quality 2: 1-9
Quality 3: 1-8
Quality 4: 1-7
Quality 5: 1-6

After Tom carefully reflected on his interviews with his three prospective practitioners, he thought, "Well, Dr. Wilson gets a '10' in competence. I'll give a '9' to Mary Smith and an '8' to Dr. Chan." He completed his chart like this:

Qualities	Dr. Wilson, orthopedics	Dr. Chan, acupuncture	Mary Smith, physical therapy
1. Competence	10	8	9
2. Interest	6	9	7
3. Access	8	6	7
4. Humor	5	7	6
5. Fees	4	6	5

4. Adding the columns will quantify your assessment of each practitioner in terms of the qualities you've deemed important. This ought to make your choice easier. Here are Tom's results:

Qualities	Dr. Wilson, orthopedics	Dr. Chan, acupuncture	Mary Smith, physical therapy
1. Competence	10	8	9
2. Interest	6	9	7
3. Access	8	6	7
4. Humor	5	7	6
5. Fees	4	6	5
	33	36	34

Close scores, of course, might suggest a combined approach. If you make this choice, be sure to discuss it with both practitioners so that they can work effectively together.

Exercise: Being Assertive With Your Doctor

In the previous chapter you read about the difference between aggressive, passive, and assertive communication styles. Here are ways they might sound (work or not work) in a doctor's office:

Aggressive: "You might have let me know about the side effects of that new medication — especially since you prescribed it on a Friday. I might have died over the weekend!"

Passive: "I'm not a doctor, so I really shouldn't say, but I've felt kind of sick from those new pills you prescribed. I guess I'm sort of a wimp, huh, for minding a little pain—but I haven't been able to get out of bed for two days now."

Assertive: "I seem to be having a bad reaction to those new pills you prescribed. In fact, I'm in serious pain and I'd appreciate it if you'd prescribe something else that might work better for me."

Recall that an assertive statement includes three features: your *perspective* or view of the situation ("I'm having a bad reaction..."), your *feelings* about the situation ("I'm in serious pain...") and your *wants* ("prescribe something else").

It's important that you be assertive with your doctor. Don't worry that this will discomfort her or him: almost every doctor I query on the subject yearns for patients to be more assertive. A typical opinion is, "Angry and demanding patients make me react in the opposite way they want. And passive, groveling ones make me just as uncomfortable, like I'm being asked to take on too much."

Try these exercises if you feel you could be more assertive with your doctor.

Visualization

1. Relax, close your eyes, and visualize yourself at your next appointment with your doctor. See yourself sitting at your full height and looking the doctor in the eye. If you happen to see yourself slouched and crumpled low in your chair, looking downward (that is, passive), or leaning forward with a tight mouth and clenched fists (that is, aggressive), alter the image until it looks simply assertive: relaxed, forthright, powerful.

2. Choose a subject you'd like to be assertive about during your next visit. Determine your perspective on the subject, your feelings about it, and the need you want met. Watch your imaginary self verbalize the three statements. Repeat them aloud. Write them in your illness journal. For example:

> I've been thinking about that operation you suggested. Considering all the stress in my life just now, I feel uncomfortable about having the operation. I'd like you to postpone it.

Role-Playing

1. Find a friend willing to role-play with you. Sit facing each other, as you would were you actually patient and doctor.

2. As an assertive "patient," enacting body language that is neither passive nor aggressive, say assertively what's on your mind. (You've given your friend no instructions how to act, so

his or her responses might actually challenge you more than your doctor's will).

You:	I've noticed that I've had to spend a little longer in the waiting room during each of my last three visits.
Friend:	(*interrupting*) Well, we've been pretty busy.
You:	When I have to wait so long for an appointment after I've arrived punctually, I feel like you don't respect my time.
Friend:	(*interrupting*) I've got a lot of patients to see.
You:	I said, 'I feel like you don't respect my time.'
Friend:	Of course I respect your time. We've just been so busy here.
You:	I'd like my next appointment to be scheduled at a realistic time. Since you have an idea how busy you are, please schedule me when you'll actually be able to see me. I'll be here on time.
Friend:	That's a good idea. I'll let the receptionist know. I'm sorry I've inconvenienced you.

Note that even though your friend interrupted, you stayed on course. And note that even though your friend initially chose not to acknowledge your statement about respect, you brought it up again. Assertiveness means holding to your honest expression until it is heard.

Exercise: Finding Your Inner Healer

You have more help than you may have realized. You have your doctor, with whom you'll continually refine your healing partnership. And deep within your imagination is an "inner healer," a subtle voice of wisdom. In this exercise you will access this inner healer, who will reveal to your conscious mind information about the meaning of your sickness and clues toward your healing.

1. Provide yourself thirty minutes of quiet solitude.

2. Sit or lie in a comfortable position, close your eyes, and fill your attention with aspects of your breath, as you did in the exercise in Chapter 1.

3. Pretend that somewhere in your body — anywhere you select — resides a profound source of benevolent knowledge, your inner healer. Begin to direct your breath exclusively into that area. Of course, you're not actually breathing into your belly or your foot; you're using the breath as a vehicle for your attention. Pretend that every inspiration gathers and focuses more attention in the area you selected, and every expiration surrenders attention directed elsewhere.

4. Sense — or pretend to sense if you need to — what feelings, what physical sensations now inhabit the area you selected. This sensation represents the presence of your inner healer. Use your imagination to develop an image of this entity. Your inner healer can be male, female, or asexual; a child, adult, or elder; human, animal, plant, or mineral; it may not even be embodied. People who do this exercise are regularly surprised by who or what represents their inner healer.

5. Illuminate your inner healer: paint vivid colors and details. Notice what facets of the image you associate with benevolence.

6. Ask your inner healer a question. Start with something simple in order to establish easy contact.

> Joan has had ulcerative colitis for several years. Her chief complaints have been occasional pain and diarrhea. She relaxes, places her attention in her breath, and mindfully moves it to the middle of her abdomen.
> ("I picked the abdomen," she says later, "because that's where my symptoms are, and I believe my colitis is trying to tell me something.")
> She feels a vague sense of movement in her abdomen. Amplified by Joan's attention, the movement

feels heavy and rhythmic.

"First I saw nothing in my mind's eye," says Joan. "But that 'moving' feeling was quite strong. I just stayed with the feeling and began to characterize it. It was a pounding sensation, like 'boom, boom, boom.' Suddenly I saw an elephant, an older male elephant who looked wise and kind. He just danced back and forth, like he'd been trying to get my attention.

"I said to him, 'Are you my inner healer?' and he nodded and smiled. I said, 'But this is ridiculous! Why should an elephant be my inner healer?' He answered, 'Well, Joan, you know we elephants might be big and ponderous, but we're quite fluid in our movements.'"

7. Ask more questions as you and your inner healer become better acquainted. Ask, for example, what are the important parts of the story your illness tells. Ask about who is significantly affected by your sickness besides you, and how these effects are manifested. Ask what you can do to heal yourself and members of your family. Ask anything you like, but understand that your answers will probably come in the form of interpretable metaphor.

Ed has multiple myeloma, a slowly progressive cancer of the bone marrow. His principal symptom is fatigue. Sometimes he can barely get out of bed, let alone perform household chores. His wife, Rhoda, has trimmed her job to half-time in order to care for Ed.

"I saw my inner healer as a duck, of all things," Ed said. "He wore a stethoscope and a nametag that said 'Dr. Quack.' I couldn't believe at first that my mind could be so ridiculous, but on the other hand, I've always had kind of a silly streak — maybe like a duck. Dr. Quack gave me a lecture about my life, showing me slides. Most of the slides were pictures of Rhoda. My God, she looked exhausted!

"I wrote in my journal that I hadn't realized how deeply my sickness affected her. We discussed it, and arranged for someone to come in and cook and clean two half-days every week. It's expensive, but not as expensive as Rhoda burning out." ·

8. Thank your inner healer with an act of kindness to yourself. The inner healer will suggest what this should be. Take it seriously. Then say your farewells.

> "My inner healer is my birthstone, an imaginary topaz," says Bert. "I consult it for healing information. When it's ready to speak to me it heats up — turns from yellow to red — and then I seem to hear words. I know there's no real topaz advising me. I just use that image as a face for my imagination.
>
> "Anyway, it told me one reason my arthritis hurts so badly was because I was lonely, which was true. My arthritis flared up something awful after Nell died two years ago. But for one reason or another, I guess I let myself *stay* lonely. The topaz said *that's* what was hurting.
>
> "I asked it what I should do about it. I mean, I don't know very many people here, and it's still hard for me to socialize. It told me just to be an ideal companion to myself for now. So I took a shower, shaved, and dressed up like I was going out on a date. Even put a flower in my lapel. I went to a great restaurant all by myself, and I must say I had a terrific time. Didn't hurt all night."

9. As usual, enter the results of this exercise in your illness journal. Include a detailed description of your inner healer and your interpretation of the healer's answers. If you'd like, ask your spouse or a close friend for their interpretation as well.

6

Your Illness and Support

Support

Support is help. It's the soil in which healing grows. Support includes physical help — such as pleasant surroundings, good food, adequate rest, and reflection time — and personal help, a particular flavor in relationships.

Physical Support

Everyone, sick or not, requires the basics: food, shelter, clean air and water, privacy, sleep, and so on. You and those who care for you need to monitor your situation to assure these necessities. Here are a few specifics concerning the major ones, food and shelter.

Eat Well

This doesn't mean eat rich or expensive foods. What I mean is this: eat nutritious foods healthily.

I'm sure you've heard the phrase, "You are what you eat." By this rule, perhaps carnivores turn fleshier or vegetarians eventually vegetate. I don't know, but I'm sure the reverse is true: you eat what you are. In other words, **your eating is invariably an expression of your self-image**.

When you feel good about yourself, you eat well. When your self-image plummets, you eat badly. This is an alarming notion, for most Americans, regardless of income, do not eat well.

People line up, engines idling, in fast-food drive-thrus to purchase "food" concocted of sugar, salt, and saturated fats, embalmed with odious chemicals, and assembled and served by disinterested teenagers who know nothing about food except that it comes in thin styrofoam containers.

At home people characteristically create meals in desultory fashion, slinging trays of highly processed stuff into microwave ovens and then, facing the TV, gobble away lest a word passes between them.

This culinary style speaks more eloquently about our national self-image than anything I might want to say about food itself. Dining can be a healing sacrament that at once honors your bodily integrity, your nurturing relationships, and the nutritive world. But all too often it is a blind biological frenzy, a herd of bipeds snuffling mindlessly in a high-tech trough.

Frankly, I'm less concerned about what you put in your mouth than how it gets there. You will generate more healing energy munching candy bars at a pleasant, congenial table than you would slurping oat bran and yogurt from your TV tray while lip-synching sitcom laugh tracks.

I suggest a couple of practices that will convert the simple act of eating into a healing event. Try these even once and I guarantee you'll try them again.

Buy real food. The most advertised foods are products so highly processed as to remove any natural texture, flavor, and nutrients. Less to be cooked than fabricated, such substances are an insult to your personhood.

Fresh fruits and vegetables, bulk grains, and honest breads, on the other hand, stimulate both senses and subtlety. They demand your creative participation. In addition, real foods cost less than industrial imitations.

Prepare the food expressly for someone you love. Do this even if you dine alone.

"When I came home after my operation," says Judith, "Max did all the cooking. He'd never cooked in his life. He brought me breakfast in bed: watery eggs, burnt toast, lukewarm coffee, and a rose. He said, 'Honey, I'd have made it better if I'd known how.' That breakfast was so good, I cried while I ate it."

Set the table. This needn't be fancy, but add an artistic flourish, like a single flower, cloth napkins, or candles. Don't invite the TV. Better yet, take your TV to the dump.

Say grace. This doesn't have to be a denominational religious ritual. Think of it literally as an act of grace, time out from everyday life. Grace is overt appreciation of nourishment and a reminder that all present pleasures are impermanent.

Take your time. Ensure that nothing rushes your meal. Excuse the kids when they'd like. Feel how life can be.

As for food itself, don't place all your faith in any particular diet. People promote dozens of diets for a given disease, and are dreaming up "New! Improved!" ones this very moment. Take them with a grain of salt. Eat sensibly (within your doctor's guidelines) while you work to perfect the pleasure and grace of your eating style.

So how do you eat sensibly? Wisdom that emerges from blue-ribbon studies seems to flip-flop weekly, so don't peg your diet to every news flash. Although the details remain controversial, however, the generalities are fairly agreed upon:

Animal fats are dangerous. Fats from animals and a very few vegetables (notably palm and coconut oil) are highly saturated fats. This means they're packed with more hydrogen atoms than are unsaturated fats, but that's neither here nor there. What's important is that saturated fats insidiously clog small arteries all through the body.

Saturated fats are by far the leading dietary contributors to cardiovascular diseases — heart attacks and strokes — and are increasingly implicated in some cancers.

That is, meat and whole-milk products are dangerous in the long run. Most commercial meat is not only high in saturated fat, but is riddled with hormones, antibiotics, and whatever else was fed or injected into the animal for marketing reasons. Smoked meats (such as bacon) contain nitrogen compounds that are known to cause cancer.

We're just beginning to realize that, like tobacco and alcohol, animal fats undoubtedly cause more deaths than heroin and cocaine put together. One day we'll probably wonder why we didn't incarcerate meat pushers.

If you're an American you probably eat too much sugar. I'm not talking about candy. I'm talking about common packaged foods. Read ingredient lists on packages the next time you shop. Try to find mayonnaise, peanut butter, crackers, or even frozen pizzas that don't contain sugar in its various euphemistic titles, such as dextrose, sucrose, and high-fructose corn syrup.

The problem with excess sugar is that it's only short-term fuel. While it makes you feel full, it supplies no nutrients other than calories. Ingested sugar not needed for immediate energy gets warehoused as fat. In 1989 surgeons performing liposuction removed 100 tons of fat from Americans. In a world half-starving, that is grotesque.

I've never understood the corporate propensity for packing sugar into almost every product. It actually shortens shelf life. And while sugar in these amounts is delicious to dental bacteria, it's relatively undetectable by consumers. Several years ago a colleague who practices medicine at a university persuaded the cafeteria's chefs to cut their baked goods' sugar by two-thirds for a week. The change apparently distressed no one, for the bakers received not a word of response from a single diner.

Eat more vegetables, fruits, and grains. It's hard to go wrong with these foods. They're nutritious, relatively inexpensive, and rich in gut-flossing indigestibles or what's known these days as "fiber."

Personalize Your Home

Your home — your house, apartment, trailer, or even cell — already says much about you. You leave evidence of your personality everywhere. An observant guest can tell, among other things, if you're sloppy, neat, or compulsively meticulous; your personal habits; your family dynamics; and your taste in books, music, and art.

Since your home expresses you anyway, what would you more deliberately have it say? Look around you in your home. What are you pleased with? Does it fairly represent who you are now? Are some elements obsolete, irrelevant, or ugly? What might you rearrange to ease movement, accommodate new habits, or enhance beauty?

Perhaps you're reading this while hospitalized. One thing that bothers me about hospitals is that they've generally been sterilized of personality, rendered as blandly utilitarian as factories.

This wasn't always so. In the Middle Ages, European hospitals were operated by the Church. The only effective medicines were spiritual: church architecture, with its mighty vaulted ceilings and radiant stained glass; religious practice, emphasizing prayer, quiet contemplation, and submission to God's will; and the grace of attending nuns. Of course, thinking at that time suffused sickness with religious concepts. Modern medicine, born with the Industrial Revolution, changed the hospital model from spiritual to secular, from church to...factory.

How you can be expected to maintain your personal spark when you've been regimented into a standard room, bed, and gown baffles me. You need reminders of your life around you. Fortunately, a growing movement in hospital administration is allowing for more individualization of hospital rooms. Patients are encouraged to bring in personal items, wall hangings, and even small items of furniture that express their presence and therefore enhance their personal power. Your insistence on important touches like these will meet increasing acceptance in the near future.

Here are a few suggestions for making your living place more of a healing place.

Learn from your home. Look at your home occasionally as an outsider might. What can you learn about the person who lives here from the way he or she apparently lives? Is this the message you wish to keep sending?

Make changes that suit your current habits. Maybe everything's fine as it is. If not, move furniture, give things away, remodel, or even consider moving. Of course, your ideas might not suit everyone, so be prepared to negotiate with family members.

Keep important mementos visible. I don't suggest this to turn your home into an egotistical hall of fame, but to encourage you to determine which memories are essential and which can stay packed away.

Display your own creations. So you're not van Gogh. Almost everyone has done a little photography, needlepoint, drawing, canning, whittling, or another craft. Honor your imagination by admitting that something you've made is at least as good as someone else's art that now decorates your home.

> "I replaced all my doorknobs and faucets with these big, bulky ones my arthritic hands can operate," says Virginia. "They're not really pretty, but they're what I need. I realized that since I'm alone now, I can do what I want, so I just keep changing things to suit me. I took out most of the furniture because the place was cluttered, and I replaced it with these big pillows. By the way, did you know I've done watercolors for years? No? Well, I doubt anyone would, since I've kept them in a closet. But now I've had them professionally framed, and I've hung them. When I get tired of them, I'll just take them down and paint some new ones."

Resist the temptation to apologize. I suppose that everyone's well-practiced in the apologetic home tour: "Please ignore the messiness." "We inherited this godawful kitchen." "We'll eventually brighten this with a skylight." "Our lawn's brown because of the drought."

Remember that your home is a metaphor for you. Since I'd advise you not to apologize for yourself, stay consistent by simply welcoming visitors without excuses. For now, it is as it is.

Personal Support

Healing can be a mysterious journey through alien territory. It's possible that you can heal without the help of others, but the process will be faster and easier with them. I once heard of an isolated surgeon who found it necessary to remove his own appendix. He did fine, but I'll bet he wished sorely for a little assistance.

People seem to mean a number of different things when they speak of personal support, so I'll offer a number of observations that I hope will make clear what it is and isn't.

Support is love. Unfortunately there are more definitions of "love" than "support." *By love I mean total attention.* You needn't entertain erotic fantasies about people or even like them, for that matter, to give them your total attention. You express your love for other people when your attention dissolves into them: you are supportive when you are free of mental chatter while with someone.

> Marty, age sixty-two, had a stroke two years ago that left him unable to speak for more than a year. He says now, "Even though my wife, Alice, had plenty to do, she spent two hours at a time with me while I recovered. She just sat with me. Sometimes she read to me. But she didn't speak much, and if you know her, you know that's not like her. We had nothing to do in those hours but just be with each other, and it was a new experience. I understand now more than ever how much we love each other. I'm speaking again, but probably less than before, and it's okay. I still love to just sit with Alice."

Support consists at least as much of listening as speaking. The most frequent question I'm asked by friends of seriously sick people is, "What do I say?" I understand their anguish. They resist saying, "Everything's going to be alright," and "I know how difficult this must be for you" because they know how vacuous these phrases can sound. They want to help, aren't sure how, and assume that their help lies in something they can say.

But the most useful support comes from *listening*, encouraging sick people to express the experience of their illness, tell you about their hopes and fears, how their lives have changed.

> "I don't know of anyone who was sick with Lyme Disease as long as I was," says Patty. "I was on my back for months while my doctors tried one antibiotic after

another. Some of my friends' help was useful to me
and some less so. One came by with some literature
and homeopathic tinctures and told me if I just followed this protocol I'd be cured. Then she left. I felt
like my sickness made her nervous.

"On the other hand, my friend Jeanne just brought
me soup now and then and usually stayed around. She
always asked me how it was for me, what it was like
to go through this. These conversations always made
me feel better, maybe because I learned from them. In
speaking with Jeanne I sometimes said things I wasn't
aware I felt."

Support is validation. When you're sick, it's hard to keep
remembering that your emotional responses are normal and significant. A supportive person is one who gently reaffirms this accepting view of your responses to illness.

"My mother has had Alzheimer's disease four years
now," says Edie. "Sometimes she's playfully childlike
and easy to be around, but just as often she's demanding and crabby. I've noticed recently that her moods
have rubbed off on me.

"My friend Rose told me she can tell how my
mother is by the way I act. She noticed that my ups
and downs paralleled my mother's. I was shocked. I
certainly never meant to be unpleasant. I began to
wonder whether Alzheimer's was contagious, and mentioned this to Rose, kind of joking.

"She told me, 'Of course it's contagious! You can't
live with someone and not absorb their moods.' She
said she'd experienced the same thing when her
father's diabetes got out of control, and that it's to be
expected. That made me feel better. At least I know
now that some of my moods aren't just me."

Support is validation of your best self. Sometimes the best
friend is the one who kicks you when you need it. The most supportive people are those who gently hold you to the truth.

Ernie recovered from major head trauma incurred in an auto accident three years ago, but was left with a permanent limp and slurred speech. He volunteers as a peer counselor at an agency for disabled people.

Today he's counseling Tom, who also slurs his speech as a result of head trauma. Ernie has seen Tom for six sessions now, and is convinced that Tom unconsciously acts in ways to put people off, especially women.

The chronic topic arises: "My problem," complains Tom, "is that I can't get women to like me. It's because of the way I speak."

Ernie answers, "Your problem is that you act like a jerk. And you talk funny. As long as you think your only problem is your speech, you'll keep on acting like a jerk."

It takes one to know one. The best help frequently comes from people who, having been where you are, can genuinely resonate with what you feel. Those who have felt their own pain and fear can more sensibly appreciate yours. For this reason the "wounded healer" is a perennially powerful notion. Some of the most effective healers I know are people who have experienced chronic or major acute illnesses.

The phenomenon of "feeling with" someone else is called in Latin "compassion." A compassionate person doesn't pity you or feel sorry for you, but simply feels what you feel. There's magic in this because you know they're in there with you.

Thomas, a fifty-year-old physician, says, "I'd never been sick or injured before. The closest I'd come was when my partner Frank had a kidney stone a few years ago, and I couldn't see then why he made such a big deal about it.

"So when I had that first attack of gout last month I realized that pain involved much more than I'd thought. I was incredibly frightened, for one thing. I was so frightened I couldn't even understand what the emergency room doctor was telling me. It was really astonishing how utterly helpless and confused I was.

"But then Frank showed up. Just seeing him brought me around, because here was a guy I knew who had hurt, too, so maybe he could understand. Frank took over my case and just talked me through it. He could tell from his own experience how lost I was, and he was able to reassure me that I was reacting normally to what was really a very simple problem.

"My patients' aches and pains look different to me now. At the risk of sounding strange, I must say that getting sick is a valuable tool for a doctor's practice."

Support begins inside. If in your core you're determined to feel hopeless and helpless — as a few people come to be — all the support in the world won't help you. You can't get pulled into the lifeboat if you don't hold out your hand.

Fred has been depressed for ten years. He's tried a variety of psychiatrists and their prescriptions, multiple courses of electroshock therapy, and various support groups, all without success. His wife, Audrey, has steadily been losing her patience, and readily angers around his problem now. At a visit with Fred's doctor, she blurted out to Fred, "Why don't you visit the burn ward and see people in real pain, people who deserve to be depressed?"

The doctor thought this was a fine idea, and arranged for Fred to visit a burn ward. Here Fred shared a waiting room with literally faceless people. He smelled necrotic flesh. He watched the agonizing dressing changes of children with third-degree burns.

"How was it?" asked Audrey. "Depressing," said Fred.

With the exception of such tenacious despondency, there is always hope. Healing is possible even where there is no hope for a cure. Under proper conditions, you can be serene even while dying. A curious but compelling notion that rings in my mind is American guru Ram Dass' advice: "I can assure you: dying is perfectly safe."

Maureen, slowly weakening with advanced cancer in the hospital, began to shriek in despair. Her doctor asked for a psychiatric consultation.

"I just saw that I was dying here, all by myself," she says. "I've always been all by myself. I thought maybe something would happen to change that, but it hasn't and now I know it won't. So my doctor sent for this psychiatrist, Dr. Sutton. I normally would have opposed that because I'm not crazy, but I gave in to it because I really didn't know what to do.

"So this lady came into my room and introduced herself as Dr. Sutton. She just stood there and looked at me. I didn't say anything. But she came over, sat on the bed, and just held my head.

"My God, I cried. And cried and cried. We didn't say much of anything at all. She cried, too, and we handed each other Kleenex. And then I stopped crying. I think I'm finished crying. Dr. Sutton comes every day and just chats with me for ten minutes, and that's all I really need now."

Recruiting Personal Support: The Support Group

Support isn't listed in the Yellow Pages. You must find it on your own. Begin with yourself, expect it from your family, and tease it out of the general population.

A powerful form of support will come from people who are in the same boat as you. If you have cancer, others with cancer — undergoing similar experiences — will be your best source of help. Let's take cancer as an example; but as you read this, plug in your own disease.

Find a support group. In my rural area we have thirty support groups for people with various chronic sicknesses, including groups for families of those with Alzheimer's disease and groups for widows and widowers.

The local branch of the American Cancer Society (Arthritis Foundation, Independent Living Center, etc.) will be happy to tell you of their own educational programs and any ongoing support groups. One of the most effective independent cancer support groups I know of evolved from an American Cancer Society "I Can Cope" course.

If there is no appropriate support group in your area, do everyone a favor and form one.

Don't expect locating other cancer patients for a support group to be easy. Word of mouth can be ineffective, as some people keep their sickness a relative secret, and personal discussion on any subject is taboo for many others. Most doctors will want to help you, but will be concerned about their patients' confidentiality.

"In some ways I guess I've always been considered an eccentric," says Ken, who has chronic leukemia. "I go see my oncologist, and while I'm in the waiting room, I strike up conversations with other patients. I usually say something like, 'What kind of cancer do you have?' I mean, only people with cancer see oncologists anyway. Most people just mutter some diagnosis and go back to reading their National Geographics. But sometimes I get into pretty good discussions.

"On the other hand, a few have complained to the doctor's staff that I'm a little forward, and that they'd rather not talk such stuff in a waiting room. So lately I've downplayed conversations and have given out my phone number. A few times people have come to my house. I'm thinking of asking them to pass my number on to other folks with cancer. I believe we might be able to get somewhere."

Despite your best efforts you may be left high and dry, with no apparent way of forming a support group. This actually happened in Sacramento, a sophisticated metropolitan area with a population of over a million, but without a visible cancer support group. A man with lymphoma wanted a group so strongly that he simply advertised in the newspaper. The ad generated enough responses to begin a group. When he eventually died, a prominent hospital offered to maintain the group.

"Carpal tunnel syndrome has been especially hard on me," says Alicia, "because I teach piano. I wanted to talk to other people who had it to see what they learned about keeping their hand dexterity. I asked some doctors and physical therapists about other patients, but they told me they couldn't release their patients' names.

"So I just put it on the radio. That's right. I found out that all radio stations are required to announce public service messages for nonprofit activities. I typed up something that looked official and sounded good. Two stations put it on the air and I got twenty responses within a week."

Any meeting of two or more people with a common interest in their sickness can be a support group. Here are a few tips for making it more than small talk:

Establish basic ground rules. Have group members agree among themselves about disclosure and confidentiality. For example, you may propose that anything may be said in meetings but that nothing said will leave the room. You may decide that certain areas are off-limits. Leave some latitude, though, for changing your mind and for issues no one has considered yet.

When Joan said, "I have faith that God will see me through this," Rosemary bristled. "I understood that we weren't going to discuss religion in this group," she exclaimed.

Steve responded, "I've been in the group since it started, and I don't remember any agreement like that."

"Well, I don't insist on speaking about religion," said Joan, "but I don't know how you can talk about life-and-death issues without it."

This led to a discussion of religion and spirituality that is still much alive two years later.

Appoint a leader. Unless someone takes responsibility for direction, the discussion can ramble into the ozone or deteriorate into stale monologues or gripe sessions. Appoint, elect, or draw straws for a leader. The position can rotate from session to session.

The leader needn't be permanent or even conversant in group dynamics. He or she is charged only with holding to the group's stated purpose and agenda. Occasionally that means assertively taking the steering wheel when a discussion seems unproductive.

> "One of the characteristics of a cancer support group is that people die," says Clair. "Let's face it — cancer is often a fatal disease. We've had four leaders in the past six years, and each one was wonderful. When Mary got sick, Nelda filled in until she got sick. When she went into the hospital, Herb took over. We've never held an election. Someone was always ready. Our leader now is Frank, who never said anything up until a year ago. But when he asked if anyone would object if he led for a while, we supported him. He's done a great job. I guess he learned it just from watching."

Determine your goals. Why are you meeting? To revive dormant miseries? Discuss the weather? Or learn from your illness and help each other to act therapeutically? It's worth spending a session exploring your purposes, for you'll be more able to conduct your meetings accordingly.

> "Excuse me, Harry," says Cecilia, who is the facilitator for this meeting of the support group for families of schizophrenics. "You're complaining about doctors again."
>
> Harry responds, "Well, what am I supposed to do when they act like pharmacists instead of psychiatrists? All they ever do is give my son pills that turn him into a zombie!"
>
> "That may be true," says Cecilia, "but we've agreed not to use this time to complain about doctors. All of us have stories to tell, I'm sure, and it's not going to get us anywhere. I think our rule is a good one. Do you want to change it?"

Harry says, "Well, it just gets me mad, is all."

"Then," Cecilia responds, "why don't you talk about being mad?"

Keep it informal. You don't need officers, by-laws, or rules of order. The closer you can make meetings resemble real life, the more useful they'll be.

"We just had our first lupus meeting in a restaurant because we wanted to keep it light," says Sarah. "You know, get acquainted a little first. But we went to the heart of the matter right away. We discussed our lupus intimately and it wasn't a problem.

"My God! The same disease affects people in such different ways! Some of them go out only at night and some don't care one way or the other about sunlight; some take all kinds of medicines and others have stopped going to doctors. I never knew I could learn so much about my own lupus by listening to other people. And I feel better knowing they valued what I had to say, too."

Make speaking optional. Remember that many people are unaccustomed to and even threatened by expressing their feelings. This gets magnified when people don't know their audience well and when they're unsure of their feelings anyway.

Assume that people who don't speak are nevertheless listening. My experience has been that people inevitably speak when they're ready.

"I knew that if I went to enough of those multiple sclerosis support groups, I'd get something out of it," says Bob, who occasionally needs a wheelchair. "Usually people in the group spoke about their feelings, and I'm kind of lost with that. Nobody's got to share their feelings with me. I've got enough of my own, thanks. But sometimes they mentioned new treatments. Last month someone said where to go for this new drug I'd heard rumors about.

"So I just went there, lived in this clinic for two weeks. When I got back and went to the group, I was

surprised people remembered me. They asked where
I'd been. I was in good humor then, even though the
medicine hadn't worked beans, so I said, 'I've got
some feelings to share. I feel like that new treatment
you mentioned a couple of weeks ago is a worthless
fraud.'"

Invite spouses. Invite spouses, roommates, lovers, primary
caretakers, or whoever happens to be closely affected by your
condition. For one thing, these people need to understand the
depth of their own involvement. For another, as you begin to act
upon fresh perspectives, the people with whom you live may be
baffled by the changes that comprise healing, and consequently
may resist them. Changes come more easily to a united household.

"Originally just Lew came to these meetings," says Jo.
"He found this group to be the best treatment for his
anxiety and insomnia after his cancer was diagnosed.
He encouraged me to come, too, but I didn't really see
what it had to do with me, and besides, I thought all
this talk about cancer would get me down even further
than I was. After a time, though, I realized I was acting more depressed than Lew, even though he was
getting sicker.
    "That made me angry. Once I even told him he
had no right to be so happy while I was miserable because he had cancer. But that didn't sound right. I said
to myself, 'Girl, you're confused. You better see what
these meetings are about.' So I came and saw how it
wasn't depressing at all. I began to get a good look at
who I was, what we were going through together, and
how to do better.
    "Lew died six months ago, but I still go to the
group every week. I learn a lot, and the conversation
here is more meaningful than almost anywhere I go."

Invite outside speakers. In most communities, specialists
offer a variety of useful approaches, including guided imagery,
physical therapy, meditation training, radiation therapy, journal-

keeping, art therapy, and so on. Usually these specialists are delighted to explain their knowledge on a volunteer basis.

> "We decided to focus on diet for six months," says Carol, the current coordinator of the arthritis support group. "There have been so many diet claims, we thought we might as well learn what we can. We assigned a half-dozen arthritis diet books to members, and they did presentations. Then we began to invite people to speak on the subject — doctors, nutritionists, and so on.
>
> "At first they talked down to us, but when they realized how much we already knew, they sharpened up. I guess word's gotten around, because when experts come to talk about diet to our group now, they act like they're speaking to other experts, and even ask our opinions."

It's possible, however, to overload the schedule with guest speakers, conveying the notion that help resides only in experts. I suggest limiting outside speakers to alternate meetings at most.

Make meetings special. Emphasize their significance by placing ritual parentheses around them. For example, you could start the group with a minute of closed-eye silence. This lets participants interrupt their daily chatter and reinforces the message that what occurs in the meeting is out of the ordinary. After all, you don't normally wear your heart on your sleeve and speak your most intimate mind. Consider ending the meeting with another ritual such as standing, holding hands, and wishing each other well.

Socialize with your group. Define occasional meetings as social gatherings without agendas. Better yet, arrange them outside normal meeting times and places. Have a Christmas party and a summer picnic. Seeing the same people in different contexts will broaden your view of them: they're not just your "cancer friends," they're your friends, period.

Eventually you may want to make a support group out of any group you happen to find yourself in. You are moving toward a lifestyle in which constant support is the ideal atmosphere.

Creating a Supportive Lifestyle

When you find that you're meeting your physical needs in a more graceful, deliberate way, and when you find that your personal contacts are likewise increasingly supportive, you may ask yourself this: can you arrange your life so that every event adds to your healing? Ideally, yes, for you always have choices.

Doctors and nurses are taught in school that each contact with a patient can potentially encourage healing. Whether you shake hands, feel organs, take blood, change dressings, or operate, you always have a choice in style. You can be impersonally mechanical or caringly present. This ideal, while not yet fully realized, nonetheless continually influences practice.

In the same way, your own behavior as a patient can be therapeutic for you. Like medical practitioners, you continually have choices. At any given moment you can take charge and decide to experiment with a different style.

But don't take the reins of your life with the expectation of future rewards; taking control *is* the reward. You can have it now. If you don't feel supported this very instant, your work is unfinished.

"I was hardening," recalls Jenny, a nurse. "I could feel it. I'd gone into nursing to help people, but all the misery and routine got to me, I guess, and a part of me turned off. I didn't want to feel people suffer anymore, so I just stopped feeling. You could say I got 'burned out.'

"When we were offered an in-service for burnout, I jumped at the chance. I saw so much in that class about what nursing had done to me and what I had done to it, I just went home and cried.

"It changed my life. I stopped covering my pain. I allowed myself to hurt, and my patients saw what I hadn't wanted them to see in the previous ten years.

"Now when I give treatments or backrubs or whatever, I feel people's pain, like I did when I was in nursing school. I've just stopped kidding myself. I really do care about people's suffering. I feel okay telling my patients that, but they tell me they already know. I'm hurting more, but I'll tell you: I'm having a better time."

Many people think of life as something that happens to them, that's handed to them; consequently they recognize their own power only in their response, never in their own spontaneous initiation.

So activate your creativity. Do something fresh and unprecedented, something that no one expects from you. Do it just to feel what it might be like to be someone different than who you've been. Write a song. Cook a new dish. Fix your own faucet. Send flowers to your spouse. Write a letter to a friend who has never written to you. Above all, notice what fresh energy feels like.

Phil had a stroke that denied him the use of language. He generally spent his days doing housework and puttering in the garden. One day his wife, Sherry, returned home from shopping and found Phil happily drawing a creditable design with a pencil. She complimented his work. Through sign language he expressed the desire for a pen.

Delighted by this unexpected interest, Sherry bought Phil a good drawing pen. He drew daily. His designs become more complex. She began to wonder where he was taking this new talent. She bought him watercolors, which he loved, and his work became even more intricate. Visitors who admired his work were given samples. Soon strangers asked if they could buy Phil's paintings. Phil was pleased, but could have cared less about selling his art: he was busy painting.

Make your life deliberate. How much of your life is either doled out to you or habitual? How much can you make deliberate?

There's nothing wrong with habits; habits are a universal source of comfort. But it's unhealthy for habits to get stale and petrified, for then you forget the element of choice involved. You begin to live on "cruise control" — an imitation of life — and that's an avoidable shame.

> "I started thinking seriously about my life right after my hysterectomy for cervical cancer when I was still in the hospital," says Amy. "People complain about hospitals being impersonal, and they are; but what impressed me was their orderliness and efficiency. Exactly what my home didn't have. When I returned home I saw — probably for the first time — what chaos our family lived in. I guess we'd just let it happen. I have no idea how the kids could have done homework in that mess or how Tom knew which socks were clean or dirty.
>
> "But no more. I announced a general, permanent cleanup. 'We're going to simplify our lives,' I said, and I've held the family to it since. Instead of mess we have order now. It's cleared my mind. I've hung art on the walls now that I can see the walls. I want flowers in the house all the time, and until my garden blooms, I'm buying them. There's no reason why I can't have a pretty life."

As you learn from your illness, you grow. Capitalize on your growth by taking your family and friends along with you. Since everyone has suffered from your sickness, why shouldn't everyone benefit from your healing as well? Teach them by demonstrating a healing life.

Exercise: Visualizing Your Support System

The first exercise is one in which you will visualize your current support and an ideal support system. You can do this exercise even if you feel that current support is lacking. Indeed, optimum support can't easily be generated unless you can first imagine its presence.

This exercise is similar to those in earlier chapters, in which you imagined things as they are now and then as they might be.

1. Ensure a half-hour of silence and privacy. Lie down and deeply relax.

2. Imagine yourself in an honest full-body view, looking as you do now. Notice detail and color in your mind's eye. Now look at the space around this image of you for images of people who currently support you.

You may or may not see your spouse, children, parents, or other relatives. You may see your "inner healer" from Chapter Five, or possibly a new figure who serves a similar role.

Now move back from this image, like a motion picture camera zooming back into a wider angle. The field enlarges. See other figures a little further from you — people who provide some support, but not as much as the primary figures.

3. What you've created is an image of your current support network as you understand it. Using your breath as a vehicle for your attention, focus this image to clarify details. Does anything surprise you? Does a particular figure seem to be more supportive than you had thought? Does a figure seem absolutely unsupportive, or even obstructive of the support of others?

4. Now, as in previous exercises, change the image into an ideal one. This may mean adding, moving, or removing figures. How would your ideal support network look? With whom do you want to be in constant contact? To whom would you refuse admission to your hospital room? Did you come across imaginary supporters you hadn't known to exist?

5. Thank your imaginary supporters personally so that your next contacts with the real people will be ones in which your appreciation is obvious. Then let your images fade. Breathe easily into your center. Memorize purely through sensation what it feels like to have your attention spread homogeneously through your body. Gradually, passively open your eyes. Sit up when ready.

6. Record the experience in your journal. Draw yourself with supporters around you. Stick figures are fine, but label them so you know which are more prominent.

7. Lead your life. You needn't push yourself one way or the other on what you learned in this exercise. You will simply find your-

self gravitating (a better word: levitating) toward people you know to be supportive.

Exercise: Setting Goals

In this exercise you will begin to create a more supportive life-style by defining short-range and long-range goals and working toward their realization.

1. Make a list of short-range goals — conceivably attainable within two weeks — that relate to yourself, your family or friends, and your neighborhood. Choose as goals events that you have desired but for some reason have put off or ignored.

For example, Elsa, a divorced woman of sixty-five with emphysema, made this list of short-term goals:

Personal: Look more interested in life.

Family/friends: Spend a pleasant day with one of my kids (closest one lives 400 miles away).

Neighborhood: Get some relief from the dogs yapping across the street.

2. Brainstorm at least three methods for attaining each goal. Brainstorming, by the way, doesn't exclude solutions that seem silly; possibilities sometimes begin as wild or illogical notions.

Here's what Elsa wrote:

Personal:

1) Get a permanent.
2) Get invited to something social.
3) Have a few friends over for dinner.
4) All three!

Family:

1) Invite daughter Sarah for the weekend.
2) Be pleasant when she comes.
3) Meet son Art half-way for a weekend (San Francisco?).

Neighborhood:
1) Plug my ears.
2) Ask a UFO to kidnap the mutts.
3) Have their owner over for tea and a chat.

3. Write a plan of action based on your brainstormed ideas. Be careful to write a feasible plan, because I'll next ask you to carry it out.
Elsa wrote:

Personal: I'll arrange to see my hairdresser tomorrow. I'll invite Earl and Dotty for dinner Saturday night.

Family: I'll invite Sarah for the weekend; she'd enjoy meeting Earl and Dotty. I'll act pleasantly with Sarah.

Neighborhood: I'll visit my neighbor, tell her that the dogs bother me, and see what she says.

4. Carry out your plan. Afterward, write in your journal what you did, what the results were, and how you feel about the successes you achieved.
Elsa wrote:

I'll admit that my perm doesn't make me into a new woman, but at least it tells people that I'm interested in how I look.

Actually, I've had a few compliments. Sarah was astonished. She said, "Mom, you haven't looked this good in years!" I just held my tongue.

Earl and Dotty couldn't make it for dinner, so it was just Sarah and me. She was so bothered by the dogs that she insisted we go together to speak with my neighbor. We did, but I did the talking. I just told her how her dogs' noise made me feel; that left the ball in her court. She was surprisingly concerned — almost mortified. They were her son's puppies, she said, and she'd ask him to come get them.

Sarah said I seemed different to her. "You're much more assertive, Mom. You're a stronger person than I

remember," she said. I think she's right. I don't think
of myself as an old shut-in anymore.

5. Now make a list of long-term goals, attainable within a few
months to a year. Their accomplishment requires the skills and
confidence you will gain from short-term successes, plus the
endurance to persist in the subtler endeavors that require a long
haul. Again, these goals should relate to you personally, your
family or friends, and your neighborhood.

Alan, a thirty-eight-year-old man with amyotrophic lateral
sclerosis (ALS), wrote these long-term goals:

Personal: Publish a book about my ALS experience that may
help others.

Family/friends: End a way of relating that neither my wife,
Roseanne, nor I like in which I passively dominate her and
and she serves me resentfully.

Neighborhood: Get wheelchair ramps installed in the shopping center.

6. Again, brainstorm at least three avenues for attaining each
goal. Alan wrote:

Personal:

1) Write a first chapter and table of contents now.
2) Speak with Lou (friend who's a published author) about
finding a publisher.
3) Research similar books in print.

Family/friends:

1) Talk with Roseanne about making changes.
2) Find a marriage counselor.
3) Maybe we can both begin watching how we behave now
and see what insights we gain.

Neighborhood:

1) Convince the shopping center's manager of the need for
wheelchair ramps.

2) Learn whether the law demands ramps, and sue if necessary.

3) Get on the city council and pass a relevant ordinance.

7. As you did with your short-term goals, write action plans based on your brainstormed ideas. Alan wrote:

Personal: I'll call Lou. Maybe he can even research similar books for me. I'll look into renting a word processor, too.

Family: I'll talk with Roseanne tonight. I'd like to go away together for the weekend and try out innovative behavior. When we get back, we can ask around about good marriage counselors.

Neighborhood: I'll call the nearest Independent Living Center (100 miles away) for advice. I'll ask Ben — a friend who's a lawyer and city council member — about the legal necessity of ramps. With this information in hand, I'll ask to meet with the shopping center manager.

8. Don't bite off too much. For now, choose one long-range goal as a project and begin to make it happen. You can always add another long-range project if you have the energy. Write in your journal weekly about what you did, what the results were, and how you feel about the progress you've made. Alan wrote:

My most urgent long-range need is to straighten out my relationship with Roseanne. Neither of us is happy with it as it is. We had a long, sometimes painful talk, and decided to have a weekend "retreat" together in the mountains.

Once there, we experimented with different styles of behaving. I was actually more assertive and she was less subservient and resentful. It was refreshing. It hasn't changed our lives much yet, but at least we see that permanent changes are possible.

We've met once with Lil, a marriage counselor, and have committed to weekly meetings for the next two months.

7

Your Illness
and Responsibility

Responsibility as Skills

You'll probably hear people speak of "taking responsibility for your illness." This advice may ring of truth, but it's a vague ring. How do you take responsibility? That is, how do you augment your *ability to respond*?

Responsibility means learning and practicing skills that aid healing. In this chapter I will discuss the most obvious ones, including assertiveness, establishing priorities, deep relaxation, and pain control.

Skills are not gifts. They require regular practice and refinement for confident use. You can hire someone to drive for you, or to play music or wash your dishes, but you can't hire someone to relax for you. Nor can you have it done by a machine or a pill. There is no way around your intense personal participation.

Every skill seems difficult at first. But think back to anything you've ever learned — typing, algebra, piano, or gardening. It probably seemed unattainable at first, but then, after you'd learned it, it was practically second nature, right? Maybe you even shrugged to novices, "Nothing to it." Keep this in mind as you practice the skills in this chapter.

Assertiveness

Assertiveness is the ability to state your mind — what you think, what you feel, and particularly what you need. Not all people can stand up and say what they need. Many of us either don't know what we need or are unwilling for a variety of reasons to express our needs.

In a previous chapter, I mentioned that if you die without a legal will, a court will dictate its own preferences for your estate's disposal. The same is true of your personal force of will: if you don't state your preferences, others will interpose theirs.

Your own assertiveness within such institutions as hospitals and even at your doctor's office will improve your care by tailoring it to your particular needs. Your ability to be assertive will also help you maintain the self-esteem that is indispensable to healing.

Increasing — and increasingly expensive — medical technology requires that institutions maximize efficiency in order to be commercially competitive. Consequently one widespread assumption is that patients are more or less standard items that can be processed identically. This isn't too outrageous: in terms of basic physical needs, one person *is* pretty much like another. Compliance with standardization can pave your road, and frequently this will be your most comfortable choice.

But sometimes you will find compliance too costly to your spirit. The assumption of standardization takes no account of the sublime, apparently infinite variations that constitute personhood. In this way, institutional policy can actually obstruct healing. There are times to be assertive.

Tim checked into the hospital to have his spleen removed as a treatment for his lymphoma.

When a staff person issued him his standard hospital gown, Tim declined. "No thanks," he said, "I brought my pajamas from home."

"You can't wear your own pajamas here," said his nurse.

"But these are my good-luck pajamas," said Tim. "They make me feel good. I'd like to keep them with me."

The nurse brought her supervisor, who said, "You'll have to wear a standard hospital gown."

Tim said, "I wasn't aware that this was such a big issue. I'll feel more comfortable here if I can wear my own pajamas. As a matter of fact, unless I'm allowed to wear these pajamas, I'll leave."

An administrator was summoned. After a short conference with her at the nursing station, the supervising nurse said to Tim, "You can wear your pajamas. But you'll have to be aware that the hospital can't be responsible if they get dirty or torn."

Tim accepted this "compromise" cheerfully.

* * *

"When Phil had his heart attack," said Louise, "the ambulance arrived within a few minutes and I rode to the hospital with him. The emergency room people stabilized him right away and arranged to admit him to the cardiac intensive care unit. He was on a gurney with tubes coming out of both arms and with an oxygen mask over most of his face. But I could see in his eyes how frightened he was.

"They wheeled him into an elevator. I followed right behind. One of the attendants said I couldn't come along, though, that this elevator was only for hospital staff. I clearly remember watching the elevator doors closing. It occurred to me that this might be my last view of him. It was like slow motion, the doors closing on Phil's eyes. Just before the doors met I lunged through the opening. It made quite a scene. The attendants looked as frightened as Phil. But I just said quietly, 'He needs me. I'm coming,' and that was that."

As you practice being assertive, keep in mind a few simple tips.

Express your feelings as exactly that. Your feelings are all you're inarguably certain of, anyway. Along California's workshop circuit, a statement about how-I-feel-when-you-do-that is called an "I" message.

So don't say, "You're a rotten, nasty creep!"
Say, "When you treat me that way I feel degraded."

An "I" message is incontestable, it puts the ball in the other person's court, and it's more likely to get the result you desire.

Take small bites before large ones. If you're unaccustomed to being assertive, don't begin by phoning the hospital administrator with a list of non-negotiable demands. Start small and locally. If your nurse leaves your teacup beyond your reach, decide not to wear yourself out stretching for it. Tell her you can't reach it. It's that simple. Every small success prepares you for a greater challenge.

Think about it first. Take the time to determine exactly what you want to say. An unintelligible roar will get attention, but don't expect things to change permanently in your favor. Imagine your ideal result before you speak.

Seek support. You may find yourself on a ward or in a nursing home where silent patients passively accept procedures and policies that strike you as intolerable. It's hard to be assertive by yourself when inertia leans thickly against you. Find support in the form of at least one other person who feels as you do and is willing to be vocal about it.

Sergio, sixty years old, awaited surgery for rectal cancer on a public ward in a large county hospital. When the doctors made their rounds early every morning, they stopped at Sergio's bed and discussed his case.

"They never discussed me," says Sergio. "They discussed my case, my cancer. They never said anything to me except, 'How you doing?' They didn't wait for an answer. Never even asked if I had questions."

One morning a professor of medicine appeared at his bedside. In a quiet, urbane voice he asked Sergio,

"Would you mind if these young doctors examined you?"

"Well, I looked at the 'young doctors,'" Sergio says. "They seemed like teenagers. I figured they must be medical students. They looked nervous and embarrassed. I said, 'What do you want to examine?' and the older doctor, he looked down at his fingers and said, 'Your rectum.'

"I said, 'You mean these eight kids are each gonna give me a rectal exam? No way, Jose!' He got pretty angry then. He told me how I was getting free treatment here so the least I could do was to help educate the students. I said, 'Doctor, I'd do it if I felt anyone here was interested in me. But I don't think they are. The house doctors are interested in 'my case' and you're interested in my rectum.'

"Well, then," continues Sergio, "the doctor got really angry and said they didn't have to treat me, that they could toss me out. That bothered me a lot. It didn't sound right. I told the nurse, and she sent for a social worker. The social worker hit the roof when I told her what had happened. She came to my bed during rounds the next morning and helped me tell the house doctors what I think and how I ought to be treated. They all looked so guilty, like someone had caught them stealing. They had known it wasn't right to treat me like I was just a rectum, just a tumor. Everything got better after that, and I never saw the older doctor again."

Learn to say no. This is one of the rarest skills in the western hemisphere. Someone must have taught us early in childhood that only ne'er-do-wells say no, for we routinely and cheerfully accept assignments that are obviously hung with skulls and crossbones.

Go to a mirror and show yourself the most attractive and pleasant face you can. Now say aloud, "No." See? No horns popped from your forehead. You're still okay. Now practice these phrases just as charmingly:

"No, I don't believe I will."

"A reason? Oh, I didn't know I needed a reason. Maybe I can think one up. For now, let's just say I don't feel like it."

"It's important to me now that I deal just with my problems, and that problem doesn't sound like mine."

"I'm sorry you feel angry/disappointed. I feel fine."

* * *

"People think that just because I look okay now that I'm as healthy as a horse, but I'm not," says Lydia. "My chronic leukemia makes even going shopping an effort. What I miss most are my weekly bridge games. Connie keeps after me to come, though, and the way she puts it, I'm letting everybody else down. I've told her every which way that I just can't do it. She told me, 'Lydia, it really makes me feel bad that of all the things to drop, you drop your bridge group.' I said, 'Connie, my own feelings are enough for me to handle; I don't have to take responsibility for yours. You're making *yourself* feel bad.'"

Once you feel good about being assertive, don't stop. You probably won't get things your way every time, but those around you will get used to hearing your preferences. If you habitually state them with neither rancor nor whine, you will come to be regarded as someone whose needs should be consulted.

Establishing Priorities

How do you order your priorities? The curse of steady good health is that your well-established routines make you forget that some things are more important than others. Illness' blessing is that the relative importance of things will become clear to you again.

When you heard about your diagnosis, this thought may have occurred to you: my days are numbered. Perhaps the initial shock bubbled off when you realized that your days have *always* been numbered. You know you're eventually going to die but until now you've been able to slide that item to the back burner.

It's time to transform your acknowledged mortality into deliberate, artful living. Select every act as carefully as you'd select dishes from the menu of a fine restaurant you'll visit only once. Here are some suggestions for developing this skill:

Notice where you waste your time. I assume from the imperfect way I lead my own life that not all your time is well-used, either. There are still a few more "nos" you could say, right? So don't take your life for granted. Look at all your behavior with a critical eye, asking where you spin your wheels, get bored, or "kill time." How much of your life is sculpted from stale obligation? What deadwood can you prune today, now?

Assume you have your "druthers" now. This very day you can go barefoot, buy a Russian wolfhound, bake sourdough rye, learn a new joke, or read to your spouse. If necessary, reread the goal-setting exercise in the previous chapter. The importance of even a tiny achievement lies not particularly in the event itself, but in what it will teach you about how to get to your next level of druthers.

Marnie is a thirty-three-year-old woman who has had a mastectomy for breast cancer. "When I was diagnosed three years ago, I had three kids under the age of five and a workaholic husband. I was a housewife, 'just' a housewife, a 'mousewife,' I called myself. I had no friends, not much married life, no hobbies, and no enjoyment. What I had plenty of was work. From before dawn I worked, doing kid stuff and house stuff until I fell over late at night.

"But the cancer and especially the operation managed to catch my attention. I said to myself, 'Look, Marnie, it might all be over soon. You have to do something about this.' I didn't know what I should do, but I knew that my life could be better. If you'd asked me what would make my life better I'd have said, 'I want to dance,' and that would've sounded silly then. Anyway, I talked to Norm about working less. He sympathized with me, but pointed out how much we needed the money.

"I swallowed that for a week or so, but then I just couldn't take it anymore. When Norm came home one night he found me packed. I told him I had to leave because I'd rather be dead than lead a life like this. He said, 'What about the kids?' I said, 'They're yours, too. Take care of them yourself or hire someone.' Well, I didn't leave. We talked for hours, and Norm saw that his easiest choice was to work less and stay home more. To hell with the extra money.

"I made sure I got out more. We arranged things so that I could go to an aerobics class every morning. I'd taught aerobics before I got married. One day the teacher didn't show up, so they asked me to teach. No problem. In fact, it was exhilarating — I thought, 'I'm dancing! I'm dancing!' When a teaching spot opened up, they asked me to start my own class. Now I'm teaching three classes a week. At least I earn more than enough to pay for childcare, and I'm meeting all kinds of interesting people! It's like my whole life opened up!"

Spend more time with people you learn from. Maybe we were all created equal, but we don't remain equal. Some folks actually glean a little wisdom along the way, and others stagger through without even noticing the pearls.

If you simply look around you in your own family and neighborhood, you'll see someone who shines, who radiates, who is literally attractive. Spend more time with such a person, because he or she is a healer for you. Learn the source of this person's glow. What makes him or her happy? What do they sense that you don't yet?

George, who was in his sixties and lived alone, finally had the back operation that he'd avoided for years. His nephew Steve, Steve's wife, Amy, and their six-year-old daughter, Justine, invited George to recuperate at their home.

George had never spent much time with Justine, but for some reason she was fascinated by George. When Justine wasn't in school, she was with George. She made him snacks, drew him pictures, and read to him from her little books.

George thought he was in heaven. "I never had

any kids of my own," he said, "because I never knew they could be like this. Justine's so innocent and loving. I never hurt when she's around."

Let go of people who drag you down. I, for one, don't need further instruction in depression, confusion, anger, and fear. I could teach a few twists to the masters. When you discover that certain people habitually emanate pessimism or depress your self-esteem, do what you can to move on. You may not be able to change them, but you can always limit your association with them.

"I was fifteen when a car accident left me paraplegic," says Andy, now thirty years old. "It took months to get back to some kind of normal routine. What helped a lot was when my parents bought me a guitar and arranged for lessons. The discipline helped me get my life back in order, and I enjoyed playing, too.

"My friends continued to visit, and they even took me out occasionally. One of them, Raymond, got on my nerves, even before my accident. He always looked at the worst possibilities. One day a few of us were playing music together. All of us but Raymond were enjoying it. He asked, 'What are those little squeaking sounds between the notes?' Typical Raymond. From that day on, I just stopped having much to do with him. Even now I weed out negativity from my life because it saps my energy."

It's harder, of course, when your millstones are family members. But there is a difference between being around sources of negativity and buying into their scheme. Deep relaxation practice may soon enable you to breathe cleanly even within a family member's neurotic atmosphere.

"When they operated on me for lung cancer four years ago I thought I was a goner," says Mildred. "I started going to a cancer support group because I was so scared of dying. I got a lot out of it — more about living than dying, as a matter of fact. My husband, Mort, would never come, though. He said, 'No use me

going. I don't have cancer.' He thought I was silly to
go, too. 'They gonna cure your cancer?' he said.

"I talked about Mort in the group. People said,
'Why do you want to be around that kind of attitude?'
I realized I was starting to feel awful around Mort, like
he was just waiting for me to die. Seemed like he already wrote me off. So I went out more with members
of the group. We went to parties and movies and such.

"Then Mort got lung cancer, too, maybe five
months ago. I've never seen anybody sink so low. He
said to me, 'How can you go out to parties when I've
had a lung removed?' The man's learned nothing. I tell
him, 'Honey, we're both in the same boat. But you're
sinking in the stern and I'm up in the prow, grinning
at the waves.'"

Deep Relaxation

How deeply can you relax? Even if your mind seems silent,
a subtle part of it continues to direct the unconscious contraction
of various muscles. You can probably hold still for a time, but
can you voluntarily soften the tiny muscles that operate your eye-
balls? How about the unwitting grip of your pelvic muscles? Can
you relax to the extent that you require less oxygen, and your
pulse and breathing rate consequently slow down?

Let's push these questions to the ultimate: how closely can
you approach being dead? I don't mean to sound macabre. I offer
the comparison as an ideal, since by definition a corpse is doing
exactly zero. Now, that is relaxation!

There's another reason I mention a corpse. When you relax
at that very profound level — and I know people who regularly
do — your mind is so quiet that everything you'd normally recognize as a marker of your personality is absent. The mental chatter that "re-minds" you of your daily dramas, your identity, your
place in your world, is temporarily gone. In relaxation at this
depth you forget who you are — your name, your sex, age, relationships, race, and even species and planet.

Strangely, though, you're conscious. Not only are you conscious, but far more aware than usual, for there is no distracting
mental chatter. It will be obvious to you at this point that as a

state of unfragmented attention, deep relaxation is less a way to check out than to check in. It's ironic that by imitating death we come so strikingly to life.

Deep relaxation happens to be a supremely effective tool for dealing with your feelings about death. Think about what people will miss when one day you finally die. They will miss who you are, your personality. But in deep relaxation your personality has temporarily departed, as though "you" have died. There you are, bereft of your individuality yet still doing just fine. The experience serves as ample food for thought. For example, is it conceivable that this broad awareness, transcending your identity as it does, survives your physical death?

Deep relaxation also serves to resolve your feelings about the self-image change that a chronic illness — and its healing — can bring about. I see this change as no less than a metaphoric death. You are a slightly different person now than you were before your illness, but you can't appreciate the change gracefully unless you let your old self drop away. Compare surrender at this level to a snake shedding its skin so that it can grow.

> Lewis learned a few forms of meditation ten years ago in order to deal with his high blood pressure. He was able to lower it enough to go off his medication.
>
> "I still quiet my mind every day, though," he says. "I learn something almost every time. One thing I've learned is that I'm more than my mind. I used to think I was Lewis, this man, this husband and father. I'm a lawyer, so I thought that's who I was, too. And a fisherman and sports car enthusiast, and so on. In a way it's all true, but getting super-quiet has shown me that these are just arbitrary envelopes around me, and that my identity can be as expansive as I choose. I've never been religious. I guess I'm an agnostic. But even so, I have to recognize what I have to call a 'spiritual' component in my life."

Exercise: Deep Relaxation

For the exercise I'm about to describe you'll need to make a tape-recording for yourself, since you can't very well keep leaving a profound relaxation to read instructions. Speak slowly and gently, spacing the recording over fifteen minutes. Play it back when you're ready to do the exercise.

After assuring yourself privacy and quiet, find a comfortable place to lie down. Deep relaxation is not the same as sleep, so diligently keep your attention present.

> Let your eyes gently close and go soft, as though they've fallen to the back of your skull. Get comfortable enough so you needn't move further. Finish with all your itches and fidgets now. Finally, lie still in comfort. The only movements remaining are those of natural breathing.
>
> [Pause]
>
> Don't change your breathing pattern. Breathe in your own style, but with each breath cycle place more of your attention in the breath itself. Sense the temperature of the air with your next breath. With the following cycle, sense the temperature along with any faint aromas. With the next, sense the temperature, aromas, and the subtle sounds of respiration. With each cycle add more sensations. Feel how one nostril might pass air more easily than the other; the movement of your ribs; the way your belly moves.
>
> [Pause]
>
> Track the air along its entire pathway, beginning with when it enters your nose. Feel it bend the tiny hairs inside your nose, course around the back of your palate, enter your throat, and descend your windpipe. Feel the air travel every millimeter of its course. If a particular area feels numb, *pretend* to feel it there, and soon you *will* feel it.
>
> [Pause]
>
> Notice how far down your windpipe you can consciously track the breath. Most people lose it somewhere in the windpipe. But now pretend to feel your inspiration go all the way down the windpipe into the center of your chest, where it divides to supply the left and right lungs. Exhale consciously from this area as well, following the air along its entire course until it's outside your nose.
>
> Everyone gets distracted along the way. Notice how your mind repeatedly conjures whatever it needs in order to pull your attention off your breath. When this happens,

don't cooperate with the distraction by getting angry or frustrated. Distraction is a normal process, and nothing to worry about. Be very gentle with yourself. Regardless of the distraction's content, persistently return your attention to your breath. It will come more easily with every practice.

[Pause]

Now pretend you can feel your inspiration flow all the way into the microscopic air sacs in your lungs, as though the air is massaging your rib cage from the inside. Soften your chest wall to accommodate this sensation. Exhale from the same place, following the breath all the way out. You are beginning to get the feeling that the flow of your breath and your use of attention are identical. Good work!

[Pause]

Over the next couple of breath cycles pretend to inhale your breath right through the bottom of your chest, into your abdomen. Soften your belly ahead of the breath. The air is not actually going into your belly, of course — your attention is. Pretend to inhale down the front of your spine, and exhale upward along the same course.

[Pause]

With each breath draw the air further down until you reach your physical center, the theoretical central cell in your body. It will be somewhere deep in your pelvis, exactly in the midline and exactly between the front and back of your body. Pretend that every inspiration collects and focuses attention at your center, and that every exhalation releases attention where it's not needed. Think of this as a process of 'centering.'

As you do this, you will probably notice a physical sensation in your center. Perhaps you will feel a buzzing, pulsation, warmth, or some other feeling. Since much normal physiological activity occurs continually in this area, a feeling here is to be expected.

[Pause]

Again, every time you notice that your mind has distracted you, either with interesting chatter, sleepiness, or boredom, return your attention gently and completely to your breath.

[Pause]

During the next couple of breath cycles amplify whatever feeling you notice in your center and expand it radially, like a starburst. The attention you have collected courses through you homogeneously, like warm butter melting through toast. You feel as sensitive in your feet as in your face. Your back is as alive as your front. You sense as much in your core as in your skin.

[Pause]

It is exclusive focus on your breath that produces this feeling of aliveness throughout your body. When you breathe in, every cell lights up. When you breathe out, every cell releases what it no longer needs.

Despite any distraction, your persistence until now means that you've probably experienced at least short periods of a quiet mind, when all there was was your breath. Notice that again now. Only the breath coming in, going out.

How passive can your breath become? Can you let your body breathe on its own, as it does when you sleep? Feel what it feels like not to voluntarily initiate the breath, not to end it, not to obstruct it, not to control it in any way. For now, regard as chatter any temptation to control the breath.

[Pause]

Now let your eyelids come open as gently and passively as possible. Let your eyes focus or not, move or not, blink or not, as they will. Notice how vision usually generates more mental chatter. When it does, return your attention to your breath.

[Pause]

Notice how you feel now, being deeply relaxed with open eyes. By deliberately sensing this passivity all through your body at once, you will memorize it so you can recreate it at will. Every time you do this exercise you will reach this level of relaxation more quickly and easily.

[Pause]

Gradually give your mind permission to distract you once again. Notice which thoughts arise first, which seem to take priority. Remind yourself that your mind is a wonderful tool, only a tool, and it is *your* tool: you are more than your mind. Congratulate yourself for accomplishing a difficult exercise. Sit up when you are ready, and return to your life.

Notice if things look slightly different to you, if the exercise has shifted your perspective a bit.

Record in your illness journal how the exercise was for you. What parts were difficult? What did you learn and what do you need to learn? How, if at all, does deep relaxation make your life look slightly different afterward?

Pain Control

"Pain" is different than "hurt."

The same level of pain can either reside in you as background music or have you writhing on the floor, largely depending upon what else is happening in your life and your attitude about what's happening. For example, I predict that you'd hurt less at your child's joyous wedding than at your IRS audit.

I'm fascinated by this phenomenon because it can help us manipulate pain voluntarily. Like other achievements I've discussed in this book, pain control can result from a deliberate shift in attitude.

Although pain is your own subjective, immeasurable experience, certain neurochemicals involved with it, called *endorphins*, are measurable. Endorphins are natural hormones, released deep within the brain and elsewhere, which are associated with pain control. Their release is triggered by virtually any analgesic (antipain drug), from aspirin through general anesthetics.

But endorphins can be released by other means as well. Some women in natural (unanesthetized) childbirth report a sudden, dramatic drop in the intensity of labor pain. At that moment endorphins can be detected in their blood. Endorphins can be found in the blood of long-distance runners who, pushed to their maximal effort, suddenly experience renewed energy, their "second wind." Endorphins can also be detected in the blood of yogis as they settle into ostensibly painful practices with apparent comfort.

This evidence suggests that we are all capable of releasing our endorphins *voluntarily*.

But these mothers, runners, and yogis are unanimous in one curiosity: they deny that their pain disappeared. They report simply that it no longer bothers them. A typical comment is, "The pain's there, but it feels like it's not me who's hurting." So in talking about pain control, I want to be clear that you're not out to obliterate pain. What you want to do is separate pain from hurt.

There are a few other things to consider before you launch into this chapter's pain control exercise.

There will always be pain. No one will ever lead a life free of pain, nor, I suggest, would that be desirable. You've probably heard the old line, "I hit myself on the head with a hammer because it feels so good when I stop." In other words, we appreciate pleasure largely by contrasting it with pain. If the whole world were only white, we would have no concept of black or, for that matter, white. Pain makes ecstasy possible. Knowledge of this principle ought to help you temper your aims.

Your pain may express your life. Even people without chronic illness hurt within unhappy situations. A century ago someone — I heard it was Karl Marx — said, "The main antidote for psychic pain is physical pain."

It may help you to know what your pain means to you — how it fits into your understanding of your life. You can regard pain as a kind of body language, a physiologically encoded, translatable message.

> Howie and Annie, in their mid-thirties, have been married eight years. During courtship they both claimed to want children, but after their first anniversary Howie noticed that Annie was obsessively meticulous about contraception. Discussing it, they both realized that Annie didn't want kids. Howie was enraged and heartbroken, but decided to stay with Annie rather than have children with another woman.
>
> Three years ago Howie's testicles began to hurt constantly. He consulted a variety of doctors, including two urologists. They examined him extensively and tried several treatments, all to no avail. Suffering increasing side effects from his prescription pain pills, Howie decided to place his attention in his painful gonads. He asked his friend Ray to listen to his images to help him clarify them.

Imaginarily inside the pain, Howie immediately saw its source. "It's a large, round steel door like a submarine hatch," he said. "It's shut tight, and it's red hot."

"What hurts in this image?" asked Ray.

"The heat and tightness are what's hurting. The door's hot because of friction, tiny things beating against it."

"Describe the things."

"Millions or even billions of things. Let's see...they're all identical. They look like little hammers, head first, handles behind. No, more like, well, rubber hammers, because the handles whip like tails. They're angry, and determined to come through that door."

Howie recorded this "story" in his illness journal and realized while writing it that it told of angrily frustrated sperm. He and Annie entered counseling.

Knowing that elements of your past can express themselves as pain, the least you can do is to avoid unnecessary grief in the present. If you're already hurting, why tempt fate by acquiescing to a current situation that you know will make you feel worse? If you're unclear about what I'm saying here, reread the section on establishing priorities and making a happier life for yourself.

By avoiding pain you perpetuate it. No one likes to hurt. You tighten your body in anticipation of pain, and when it arrives you squirm away from it like a hooked fish. You fill your mind with desperate denials ("I can take it"), gobble pain medicines, and maybe even opt for palliative surgery.

These attempts are usually successful in the short run, and for the short run I heartily recommend them. There are few greater joys in medical practice than giving intravenous morphine to someone screaming with kidney stone pain and then watching his grimace change to an easy smile.

But when pain becomes a chronic companion, short-term solutions backfire.

Denial actually highlights the pain. Telling yourself, "I refuse to recognize this pain," you have perpetuated its presence. Try this now: refuse to think of a purple elephant. See what I mean?

Chronic use of pain medicines diminishes your ability to release your own endorphins. That is, you will come to require more and more pills while being less able to control pain naturally. Furthermore, you will get sick if you stop taking the pills. We call this addiction. And pain-oriented surgery is usually "iffy," as your surgeon will attest.

So if you find the traditional approaches to your chronic pain wanting, try doing the opposite: put your attention *in* the pain, as in the exercise I'll soon describe. Note that I didn't say, "Put your attention in the hurt." By fully appreciating the pain by itself, without emotional filters, you will discover, along with the mothers, runners, and yogis, that pain doesn't need to hurt.

You can control some degree of pain. Look around you and you'll see that all individuals have their own "pain threshold," the amount of pain they'll take before seeking help. You have your own threshold, and your past experience will reveal that it has varied from time to time. Since you've already controlled pain to some extent, even inadvertently, consider it time to enhance this ability as a conscious skill.

Aim for a target you can hit, between what you already know how to do and some ultimate limit. Use the following exercise — an extension of the one at the end of Chapter 2 — to push your present capability. Your developing skill in voluntary pain control will eventually come to supplant at least part of your medical antipain regimen.

Exercise: Pain Control

1. Assure yourself twenty minutes of solitude. Lie in a comfortable position. Quiet your mind. Relax as deeply as you learned to do earlier in this chapter.

2. When maximally relaxed, direct your attention into the area of your pain. Begin to regard it as just another sensation rather than as "pain." Use inspiration to "breathe into" the area and exhalation to surrender any attention held elsewhere.

3. Be respectful and gentle with the sensation. Don't go to its imaginary center immediately. Gradually spiral in from its periphery.

4. As you did in the exercise in Chapter 2, begin to characterize this sensation you've called pain. What does it feel a *little* like? What does it feel *more* like? Progress toward what it feels *exactly* like. Remember, you're translating a feeling into an image as accurately as you can. And since the feeling has an unpleasant aspect, find that aspect in the picture.

> Helen got severe headaches at work almost every Friday. She wouldn't take pain medicines, and a variety of therapies made little difference. She tried this imagery exercise.
>
> Having deeply relaxed, Helen almost lost the headache entirely. Just enough remained for her to work with. She compared the feeling to a clamp around her head. She refined the clamp image to a vise pressing her temples. It was plain to her that the pressure represented her headache.

5. Change every unpleasant aspect of the pain image until the result looks ideal. Again, you're limited in this work only by your imagination. The change in image will almost always alleviate the pain significantly and quickly. Once you achieve an ideal picture, illuminate it vividly so it becomes an influential memory.

> In her mind's eye, Helen interposed her own hand to open the vise. This didn't work. She attempted to turn the vise into a soft, cool washcloth, but it didn't want to do this, either. Finally it occurred to her that the vise might be brittle, so she simply punched it with her fist and indeed it disintegrated.
>
> As the vise fell away, she looked closely at her temples. They seemed pale and depressed, so she "breathed" some pink into them. She zoomed back to see her whole head. She looked happy, healthy, radiant. She was sure she'd remember this image.

6. Let go of the image. Let it fade. Return full attention to your breath as you sense throughout your body the feeling of deep relaxation. Let your eyes open passively. Slowly sit up, resuming your everyday consciousness.

7. Enter the entire story in your illness journal and follow it with an interpretation. If you'd like, have your spouse or close friend comment on it as well.

> Helen wrote: "A clamp around my head became a vice (how do you spell that?) around my temples. I tried to open the vice with my hands, but couldn't. Tried to change the vice to a soothing washcloth, but that didn't work either. I finally broke it off and made my head look alright again.
>
> "What does it mean? It's hard to forget the trouble I'm having with David. My family opposes us living together and we're not getting along well, anyway. They're pretty conservative. They say premarital sex is a...vice. And they don't like me seeing someone outside my religion. David is an orthodox Jew. Is that why my 'temples' hurt on Fridays? Are my headaches telling me to 'break it off'? I have to talk with David about this."

In Case You Forget...

You needn't memorize everything in this chapter. The main thing to remember is that these skills all have a common focus: your attention. An excellent way to develop your attention is by practicing deep relaxation. By definition, when you've placed all your attention in aspects of your breath, there's no attention left for such distractions as pain, stress, or other elements of the compelling drama we know as illness. So if no other skills come easily, focus on deep relaxation.

8

Your Illness and Transition

Transition

A sure bet in the chronic sickness lottery is that things will change.

The disease will get better or worse, and meanwhile your life with all its variables will go on until you eventually die. In addition, every change will affect those around you. I want to use this final chapter to promote graceful transitions and to introduce a perspective that aims toward illness prevention.

Progressive Sickness

Think on this: barring sudden death, everyone will get progressively sicker. As always, what's mostly unpleasant about this prospect isn't the condition itself but your fear of it — and *that's* something you can deal with.

Abrupt catastrophes, such as the accidental loss of limbs, mental faculties, or loved ones, can generate disturbances that take years to recover from, if recovery occurs at all. But the same losses incurred over longer periods — as in chronic sickness —

become more tolerable. I've seen people who choke at the thought of becoming dependent on others, for example, accept dependence peacefully when the process is gradual.

Here are some ways to accommodate more gracefully to your chronic disease's slow evolution.

Take one day at a time. I borrowed this slogan from Alcoholics Anonymous because it works. Changes that accumulate without your recognition will eventually reach a critical mass that can be shocking. For example, a loss of twenty pounds will decimate you if you refuse to look at yourself more often than every two weeks. But if you consult your mirror daily, the continuity will make the change more acceptable.

In addition, you may notice unexpected upswings that would have remained hidden had you decided to withdraw your senses.

> Sick with advanced cancer, Selma had been taking sizable doses of morphine. Suddenly she stopped asking for it. "I hadn't expected this but there's actually less pain now," she said. "I can handle this alright. I'd rather be mentally clear to feel what happens as I die.
>
> "It's funny how this works. I was so worried about getting cancer, and then I got it and learned to live with it. Next I worried about getting disabled. But the cancer advanced a little at a time, so here I am disabled as can be, and doing okay. I guess I've learned I can handle whatever comes my way. There's nothing more for me to fear, so I'll just lay back and watch."

If you're able to, write daily in your illness journal, simply to check in. Write how you feel today and how you feel about the progression of your sickness. Share any revelations from your diary with people around you so that they can keep up, too.

Do what you can. Enact your maximum capabilities — however attenuated — day by day, or hour by hour, if necessary. After all, you're still leading your life.

> Jake's neurological disease progressed to the point where he found it hard to get out of bed. Occasionally

he needed mechanical help breathing.

"If it weren't for that one step forward in between the two steps back, I think I'd throw in the towel," he said. "I learned to treasure a few minutes walking without help, and now I treasure a few minutes with my walker. I guess soon I'll look forward to breathing on my own. It's been important all through my sickness to challenge myself, and I can almost always find a little reserve I hadn't expected."

Discuss all possible medical interventions with your doctor in detail. Minimize the possibility of unpleasant surprises. Does your doctor contemplate intravenous feeding? Mechanical breathing support? Organ transplants? What are your wishes in regard to artificial life support if you become comatose? Do you wish to have your name added to an organ donor directory? When you die — when your pulse and respirations cease — do you wish resuscitation attempted or not? Ask what your doctor will do in case legal documents you generate on these issues are not sustained by a court.

Discuss ramifications with your lawyer as well. Draw up two indispensable documents, a will and a *durable power of attorney for health care.*

If you don't say what you want done with your estate, a court eventually will. "Eventually" can mean years. For everyone's peace of mind, a current will is a necessity.

A durable power of attorney for health care allows someone you trust to make binding decisions for you if you cannot. Suppose, for example, you were to become comatose or irreversibly brain-dead. You might have chosen to decline mechanical life support, but being perforce incommunicative at the time, you wouldn't be able to state your preference. This document — which you should prepare with the help of an attorney — allows the person you choose to make decisions in your behalf. Provide a copy to your doctor and to the hospital for permanent residence in your records.

Surrounded by his wife, Elaine, and his children, Marvin was seriously sick in the hospital. Marvin had always considered any talk of dying distasteful, so had neither discussed it nor developed any relevant legal documents.

Finally Marvin sank into a coma deep enough to require a breathing machine. Elaine sent for the rest of the relatives. She also requested Dr. Cargill to cease artificial support once the relatives had said goodbye. He responded that because of legal liability he could not comply with her request.

By the time the relatives arrived, Marvin could once again breathe on his own. In a few hours he was lucid. He recognized his visitors and spoke to them weakly but intelligibly. When Dr. Cargill asked him what he'd like done if he became comatose again, Marvin said he'd rather not talk about it — that Elaine and the doctor could decide. Dr. Cargill explained that if Marvin himself didn't make these decisions, he, the doctor, would be bound exclusively by the hospital's policies. Nevertheless, he couldn't persuade Marvin to make the decisions.

Marvin fell into a coma again that evening. As Elaine voiced her opposition, Dr. Cargill once again put Marvin on life support. A few relatives disagreed with Elaine, and soon the family fell into a bitter dispute that dredged up decades of grievances. Marvin's heart suddenly stopped. Resuscitation attempts were unsuccessful. Elaine's introduction to widowhood unfortunately began amidst heated family dissension.

* * *

Eldon, long sick with cancer, became comatose. Following their standard procedure, the hospital's staff put him on mechanical life support. A social worker contacted his next of kin — Marge, Eldon's estranged wife — in a nearby city.

Marge was furious that Eldon was being kept alive artificially. "He hated gadgets like that his whole life! He wouldn't be caught dead with one!" she told the social worker.

The social worker patiently explained that indefinite life preservation was this hospital's policy. Two hours later Marge showed up at Eldon's bedside with a valid three-year-old durable power of attorney for health care that gave her the right to make decisions. "Please let him go," she instructed, and her wishes were followed.

Healing

As I discussed earlier, you may heal regardless of any course your disease takes. Healing means that in some degree you become a different person. But no one changes in a vacuum. The various consequences of your illness pervade the habits and emotions of those around you.

I explored social ramifications of illness in Chapter 4, but postponed until now a discussion of the effects of your healing on others.

Believe it or not, your healing may not be greeted with a tickertape parade. Suppose those around you have already adjusted, with great effort and difficulty, to the idea of your chronic illness or death. In their new mental set they may expect you to behave in a particular way. Imagine, then, what even slight physical or attitudinal recovery will do to others: you may appear suddenly alien and therefore threatening. Your improvements may throw them into psychological turmoil all over again.

If this happens you'll have three choices. You can back off from your changes in order to assuage others' anxieties; you can decide to push on and leave those other folks behind; or you'll do what you can to bring them along.

Anna has been paraplegic since having polio at sixteen. Now in her forties, she's married and has two teenagers. "Five years ago I dreamed I was out of my wheelchair," Anna recalls, "walking, while a huge bird soared above me. The next day a friend introduced me to a faith healer named Jim, who has a picture of an eagle on his business card.

"So I saw Jim for treatments. By the third treatment I was walking! Oh, it wasn't very graceful and I needed two canes, but I was walking.

"When I showed my family I could walk, they were horrified. 'Sit down, mama! You'll fall and hurt yourself!' my kids said. My husband said, 'But we're already used to you in your wheelchair.' Anyway, the easiest thing for me to do was to get back in my chair, and there I've stayed."

* * *

"I don't know what's come over Lana," says George. "Ever since that cancer operation she's been snapping at me. Is that a part of cancer?"

"What George can't seem to understand," Lana comments, "is that I'm different now. He doesn't see it. But my time is more important to me now, and I'm not about to put up with his old crap anymore."

* * *

"Ever since Margaret and I divorced," said Jim, "the boys have tried to manage my life. I don't know where they got the idea I can't run a home myself. They both have their own families just a few blocks away, but it seemed like they were always over here, cooking and cleaning and fixing.

"When I got sick, their help was a godsend. But while I convalesced, I got clear on a few things. I discovered I really don't want them around so much. Actually, the boys have a little problem depending on me. They needed to help me for their sake, not mine. Maybe this whole pattern began in their childhoods, but at any rate it's not healthy now.

"I spoke to them about it gently. I didn't want them to take it wrong. Art, the older one, has been in counseling a while, and it's something his therapist had already suggested to him. Anyway, a few discussions persuaded them. Now they help when I ask them to, and it's really satisfactory."

It's always nice to bring loved ones on any journey. If you're benefiting from what you've learned, why shouldn't they? Here are suggestions for pulling them aboard.

Keep them informed. Don't hide the details of your healing from others or, for that matter, from yourself. Consult your illness journal daily to comprehend your perceptual shifts. You might be experiencing more rapid change now than at almost any time in your life, so try to express yourself as it happens. Sometimes understanding will come to you only as you articulate the situation.

Mindfully enact what you've learned. Unless you act it out, as a matter of fact, you haven't learned. People will definitely notice: healing is subtly contagious. Those around you can ease their own passage through life simply by absorbing your example.

Don't feel guilty about changing. You're not demonstrating fresh perspectives for the purpose of making anyone else's life harder. Consider instead that you're favoring others by showing them what a more positive attitude looks like.

Dying

Since death doesn't have an easily definable beginning and end, the word "dying" has questionable application. As I mentioned in Chapter 1, you don't know someone is dying until he or she has died. Only then can you say confidently, "That person was dying."

Still, there are often signs of impending death. Moribund people get weaker. Their consciousness diminishes or disappears. Their vital signs — pulse, respiration, blood pressure — become slim and erratic. But these signals appear rather shortly before death. What are we to say of the weeks or months that precede them?

Until you die, you are incontestably living. Notwithstanding your symptoms, your personality makes itself known. You eat, sleep, and relate in your fashion, and this, for now, is your life. Make the most of the moment, for you won't be back this way again. Don't decide to withdraw yourself from those around you based on the notion that you're dying. Actual dying requires no decision on your part.

> "I've had four heart attacks now," said Barbara, age seventy. "Each time the doctors save me, but a little more of my heart dies. Now it doesn't pump all the blood that comes to it, so my legs are swollen and I

have fluid in my lungs. I have to sleep sitting up, or else I can't breathe. The doctors have as much as told me I'm dying.

"So I don't make many plans, but at least I don't just sit around and wait to die. My son got my needle-point materials out of storage, and I've been finishing all those old pieces I said I'd get to one day. There's really nothing I'd rather do."

Life as Transition

Transitions such as sickness and death — and sometimes even curing — can be hellishly inconvenient. We want our lives to be simple yellow brick roads with a clearly labeled beginning, middle, and end. The zigzags and backtracks that constitute real life can look at first like unjust intrusions.

"Sam went into a coma right after I said goodbye to him," said Christine. "We were expecting it. One of the doctors told me that Sam probably didn't have more than a couple of days at the most. The family said goodbye to him, made funeral and memorial arrangements, and began to think about what life would be like without him. I was going to sell the house and move to Arizona.

"I stayed at Sam's bedside for two days, three days, a week. Nothing changed, so I began to come every other day. I felt like I couldn't do anything definitive while he was alive. I started staying home more than visiting Sam, but when I was home I just watched TV or sat around depressed.

"That was two months ago. My family and friends can't do anything for Sam, and they probably feel they can't do much for me until Sam dies. He's still in a coma. The doctors and nurses are getting food and liquids into him, and I'm not about to ask them to stop. But his lingering has really disrupted everyone's life. I've even found myself angry with him sometimes, and that doesn't make me feel good."

Curves, detours, and dead ends *are* the path. Life is built entirely of transition, of which sickness is just another example. Life is a cradle-to-grave parade of change, the antithesis of consistency.

Seeing sickness as separate from life or larger than life will inflate it beyond your ability to cope.

So begin to see transition everywhere, for that is the incontrovertible state of things. Sorry, but diamonds are not forever. Within a cosmic time sense, the earth was once and will again be spacedust, and we're here for a gnat's eyeblink. Like it or not, we are citizens of time, and time is identical to change.

Yet we understandably conspire to maintain an illusion of stability. Indeed, that illusion is a requisite of culture itself: without it we wouldn't recognize our homes or each other, and our language would be unreliable from day to day. So we act for convenience as though time is a ratcheted progression of static realities. But it is not: it flows smoothly, seamlessly.

If you yourself are anything, you are change. Pretend to photograph someone's entire life with a time-lapse camera, compressing it into a minute. What you see is the union of sperm and egg, a growing fetus, an infant, child, adult, a gradual shrinkage to senescence, and finally decomposition. If this were a film of your life, which frame would be "you"?

You continually shed cells of the skin and gut and replace them with fresh recruits. Specialized cells labor night and day to resorb existing bone and lay down new bone. You have none of the red blood cells you had four months ago. Today's neurochemicals are tomorrow's urine. It's said that your cellular makeup turns over completely every seven years or so.

Yet you nevertheless retain a concept of "you." So do I. This sense of continuity is a useful mental construct, but never a property of flesh. You might approach a more reasonable self-image if you consider yourself a process instead of a "thing." Take Buckminster Fuller's notion seriously: "I seem to be a verb."

If you do, sickness will begin to look less like a horrid disaster and more like a natural — however difficult — part of your life. The better you accept this transition we call sickness, the better you will respond to it.

"I don't have to be who I was," said Janet at a cancer support group meeting. "The only thing that holds me to my past is my attitudes. Change those, and I change who I am now. Since I got cancer I've changed more attitudes than I ever knew I had. At what point can I call myself a born-again human?"

* * *

"I used to think my spastic colon came on suddenly, like a heart attack," said Nikki. "But working with my therapist, I've recalled symptoms as far back as my memory goes. So is my condition something I suddenly 'caught' or something that is part and parcel of my entire identity?"

Learning Without Sickness

So far I've encouraged you to see your sickness as meaningful. If you applied the foregoing principles fruitfully, you may now view it easily in that context. You may now feel as though your sickness is a long-overdue opportunity for growth. Or perhaps you see your cure as preparation for your destiny, or your eventual death as a mandate to get your wheels into gear.

Good! But I'll encourage you in this final chapter to flip around and regard sickness and its consequences as nothing special.

I'm not degrading the importance of your sickness. On the contrary, I'm asking you to elevate other events to an equivalent status. This is feasible, after all, since significance is arbitrary: you simply assign it where you like.

By seeing significance in more events — whether or not they're related to sickness — you'll reap lessons. That is, you don't need to get sick in order to learn. *Learning without getting sick is the ultimate preventive medicine.*

Lessons surround you, waiting only for your recognition. Once you realize that your most creative response to burning your toast requires the same attitudinal tools that can help you die gracefully, your kitchen mishap will mutate into a valuable opportunity for practice.

The key to this discipline lies in creating adventure, developing a personal alchemy in which the mundane is redefined as the extraordinary. Here are a few suggestions for doing this.

Take less for granted. Since your mind will chatter anyway, make it do so artistically by having it read significance into more events. Doubt coincidence and randomness.

I'm advising you to be a scientist, not a mystic. The history of science is essentially a search for patterns. Our most revered scientists are those who seek patterns of patterns. Said Einstein, "I want to know God's thoughts. The rest is detail."

One thing we know about life is that it doesn't come with an instruction book or a guided tour. Your interpretation of an event is simply that: your interpretation, a product of your mind. That is, what you see is largely who you are. Looking outward with deliberate intelligence is a way of looking in.

If you can read meaning into a sickness, you can read meaning anywhere — and act on it. After all, wouldn't you rather respond today to the caress of an existential feather than next week to a blow from a two-by-four?

"I found a badly injured dove flapping her wings on the road," said Betty. "She'd been nicked by a car, and it looked like she was dying. I'd never stopped for a bird before. I picked her up and carried her to the side of the road, sat with her, and patted her until she died. As I sat there I thought about her innocence and vulnerability; then it occurred to me that I was really thinking about myself.

"I'd been diagnosed with lupus three months then. At that point I had no symptoms and was on no medications, so I thought I was tough enough to continue my life as it had been — job, family, and all. But my experience with the dove showed me that I need and deserve protection. So now I plan to take better care of myself. I don't have to be tough. I've begun to talk with my husband about how I'm going to cut back and get more rest."

* * *

Theodore was certain that his chronic headaches were related to his executive position. "It always felt like I'd never done enough," he said. "I considered my reports to my boss inadequate — even though they got fine evaluations — and I felt like I continually let my subordinates down.

"But at home I always felt guilty, too. Hardly ever helped with housework, not there enough for the kids, gave too little to charities, that kind of thing.

"One day I came across one of the kid's stuffed animals in the backyard. It was waterlogged from rain, and had almost come apart. My first thought was that somehow it was my fault the toy was ruined — as though I should've found it earlier or disciplined the kids better.

"But suddenly that stuffed animal looked like something else, and that something else, I realized, was my waterlogged mind. I saw that I characteristically projected guilt onto whatever happened in my life — good, bad, or indifferent.

"I checked this out with my wife and a friend, and they confirmed it. In fact, they both said they'd already told me this repeatedly, but I'd never been able to hear it before.

"Now when I feel guilty I challenge myself about it. I say to myself, 'Is that stuffed animal there again?' My headaches, by the way, have almost entirely disappeared."

Have an adventure. Without adventure you'll slide into the quietly desperate style of predictably choosing present miseries over every unknown future.

An adventure doesn't have to be a Caribbean cruise or a barrel-roll over the falls. Any event can be stimulating, depending on your attitude. Seen anew, everything sparkles with possibilities.

Jack fell off his roof and broke both heels. "I was in two casts for months," he said, "completely disabled. So I just sat on my easy chair and read, mainly. It wasn't so bad, since I'd been laid off work and wasn't looking forward to going out into the job market. In fact, after my casts were removed, I still just sat and read.

"My friend Larry dropped by once in a while, and he got concerned. One day he said, 'Jack, you're melting away here. You need a little action.'

'What do you have in mind?' I asked him.

'Well, let's go for a ride.'

'Naw, I'd rather sit here and read.'

"But he talked me into it. He drove me up to that ridge behind town and made me look out to the horizon.

'You already know where you're at,' he told me.

'Now it's time to look at all the places you can go to.'

"I took Larry seriously, and it was an amazing experience. I began to think in whole new ways, actually considering my personal horizon. That was five years ago. I've moved since then, and got a good job. I don't think everybody needs to drive up a mountain, but it sure helps to do something that gives you a wider view."

Experiment with your personality. You're only as petrified as you believe you are. It's difficult, though, to try out new behavior at home, since those familiar with you expect your habits. So first try going away where no one knows you and consequently has no expectations.

"I figured that as long as my arthritis was going to hurt anyway, I might as well be in pain in pleasant surroundings," said Doris. "I took a bus to that hot springs resort I'd heard about.

"I soaked in hot water the first day and in hot mud the next. All that time I was surrounded by other arthritic widows complaining about their arthritis. I thought to myself, 'Wow! No one knows me here. I'll try out a different Doris and see what it feels like.' Well, for three days I chose not to complain. Not one complaint, grimace, or wince. Very unlike me, right?

"I met some very lovely people. Since I didn't complain or even discuss my arthritis, they all assumed I was guarding some great health secret, and began asking me for health tips. I came home feeling great!"

If you're successful with this experiment away from home, try it again when you return.

"It feels like I've been angry forever," says Mark, age thirty. "I don't know why. I've seen shrinks and combed through my childhood and all, but I've stayed angry.

"I've been meditating for years now. I'm gradually getting good at it. Several months ago my teacher asked me, 'Mark, why don't you use meditation to see what you'd be like without your anger?'

"Well, that had never occurred to me, so I tried it. I learned I could just sit and be conscious without anger. I liked being angerless Mark! I can produce that feeling at will now."

Continually reevaluate what is important. Do features of your life that you called important yesterday remain as important today? A fresh look may reveal that you've spent undue energy on trivia while ignoring what deserves greater prominence.

"Before Linda got sick," says her husband, Byron, "we had fairly routine lives. Work, shopping, menus, kids' schoolwork, and so on. After she got sick we held to those same routines. Maybe that helped us keep our sanity for a while, but it got out of hand, living as though she wasn't sick.

"She got weaker, I got more exhausted, and then we just had to face reality. I suppose we'd been in what people call 'denial' about her sickness. Did that change what we did? You bet! We know now that what's important is loving each other and taking care of each other. All the daily routines are nothing compared to that."

The Spiritual Dimension of Transition

I predict that the 1990s will be the decade in which spirituality comes out of the closet. It has languished so long that spurious notions have grown on it like mold. Some people link spirituality with negative memories from childhood religious training. Others see it as an anachronism in our modern scientific world, or perhaps have heard about it mainly from people whose feet don't quite touch the floor.

But properly understood, spirituality is to healing as wings are to birds. My challenge is to describe spirituality in terms that will be practical and ecumenically acceptable, even to hard-nosed scientists.

"Spiritual" Means Expansion of Your Sense of Self

How large a self-image can you inhabit? Do you act from within a few exclusive categories such as your gender, age, and social status? These local, limited self-images are certainly honest, accurate, and useful; but remember that they degrade and die with your body. To the extent that you confine your self-image to these categories, your healing potential is limited.

You may choose to see yourself more inclusively, transcending your age, gender, race, and nationality ("human being"); transcending your species ("earthling"); or even transcending your galaxy ("child of God," "sentient being").

You needn't abandon your smaller identities to appreciate larger ones, any more than you'd discard short screwdrivers after buying a long one. Smaller identities are valid descriptions, and most daily activities require cultural conformity. But other endeavors — such as healing — might ask more of you.

> "Before I got cancer," says Kate, "I was pretty sure who I was: a woman, a wife, a mother, a daughter, a teacher. But my sickness diminished me. I found myself less wife and mother, for example, and totally unable to work as a teacher. In fact, I began to wonder what would be left of me if all my identities dropped away. This bothered me a lot. I thought I might literally become what used to be called an 'invalid,' which to me means 'not valid.' This fear bothered me more than my cancer symptoms did.
>
> "With the help of a meditation teacher, I've learned to quiet my mind to the extent that every

reminder of who I am *does* disappear; I'm fully conscious without any of my personality present.

"It's paradoxical: by letting go, you get. I'm not sure I believe in reincarnation, but I've experienced a strong sense that something about me will survive my eventual death. There's much more to me than flesh."

Exercise: Your Spiritual Identity

1. In your illness journal, make a list of ten identities that describe you. Create columns labeled A and B on the other side of the page.

Dave, hospitalized many times with sickle-cell anemia, wrote this:

Identities	*A*	*B*
1. Man		
2. Father		
3. Son		
4. Husband		
5. Brother		
6. Afro-American		
7. Baseball player		
8. Follower of Jesus		
9. Sickle-cell patient		
10. Salesman		

2. In column A, place an x opposite each identity that will die when you do.

Dave filled in his chart this way:

Identities	*A*	*B*
1. Man	x	
2. Father	x	
3. Son	x	
4. Husband	x	
5. Brother	x	
6. Afro-American	x	
7. Baseball player	x	
8. Follower of Jesus		

9. Sickle-cell patient	x	
10. Salesman	x	

3. In selecting those identities that will die when you do, there were probably a couple that you wondered about. Go over the list again, and put an x in column B for those identities that you feel might in some way survive your death. Explain these in your illness journal.

Dave filled in his chart this way:

Identities	A	B
1. Man	x	
2. Father	x	x
3. Son	x	
4. Husband	x	x
5. Brother	x	
6. Afro-American	x	
7. Baseball player	x	x
8. Follower of Jesus		x
9. Sickle-cell patient	x	
10. Salesman	x	x

Dave wrote, "I guess I've been average in some ways, but I've stood out here and there, too. People will remember me as a really good father and husband, a terrific baseball player, and a hell of a salesman. After I die, those memories of me might be strong enough to live on in my place. And I know I'll always be a follower of Jesus, living or not."

4. Consider the items in column B. What is special about these identities? What qualities have you brought to them? How have they expressed the best part of you? Why does it seem that they might somehow survive you?

Dave wrote: "Looking at column B, I recognize that what will live after I die are the things I loved doing. What made me a good father was what made me a good husband, ballplayer, and salesman. I just loved doing them all, and I guess it showed. What I'll really leave behind, then — and take with me, too — is love."

Medicine's Transition

I was informed in medical school that the whole is exactly the sum of its parts — not one iota greater — and was then trained in great detail about all the parts.

People are DNA-programmed biochemical gadgets, we were taught; imagination is an illusion generated by brain biochemistry; life happens meaninglessly; sickness, the curse of an unconscious universe, randomly afflicts innocent, passive victims; and medical treatment consists of jimmying disordered molecules back into working condition.

This philosophy is internally consistent and powerful toward its own goal — renovating errant physiology. In addition, it is incomplete: it ignores the poor soul who experiences the sickness. This state of affairs continually leaves patients *and their doctors* unfulfilled. I don't believe this sad situation is a medical conspiracy. It's more serious than that. It is, in fact, a problem that pervades western culture.

So I've departed from the philosophy in which I was trained. Now I practice as though life is a stream of choices; as though imagination is real, not imaginary; as though people are necessarily involved in their sicknesses; as though illness is wisdom wrapped in pain. And if indeed we are biochemical gadgets, at least we're gadgets capable of great power and love.

I'm not alone in this. Medical practitioners and patients *en masse* are coming to similar conclusions. After 250 years, we're finally freeing ourselves from the iron grasp of the Industrial Revolution. We are striding toward a balance of technology with humanism. We are entering an age of passionate exploration of the mystery that is us.

At last we can ask publicly, as scientists, the questions that haunt our hearts. Is any event random, accidental, or coincidental? Where were you before you were conceived, and where will you go when you die? Can your mind operate outside your body? What, for that matter, is the body-mind relationship? What are the subjective factors that can create and treat sickness? Is there an end to healing?

Further Reading

General

Carlson, Richard and Benjamin Shield, ed. *Healers on Healing*. Los Angeles: Tarcher, 1989. (Essential reading; forty well-known healers in various disciplines illuminate the themes common to all.)

Cousins, Norman. *Anatomy of an Illness*. New York: Bantam Books, 1979.

_____. *The Healing Heart*. New York: Avon, 1984. (Profoundly empowering explorations of the personal aspect of sickness.)

Dossey, Larry, MD. *Beyond Illness*. Boston: New Science Library, 1984. (Well-reasoned treatise that says, basically, that sickness is a normal human phenomenon and possibly even a learning experience.)

_____. *Meaning and Medicine*. New York: Bantam Books, 1991. (Fascinating discourse on the interpenetration of meaning and illness, documented by respected medical research findings.)

Illich, Ivan. *Medical Nemesis*. New York: Pantheon, 1982. (Cynical but faultlessly documented history of modern medicine's increasing dangers and arrogance.)

Jampolsky, Gerald, MD. *Love Is Letting Go of Fear*. New York: Bantam Books, 1985. (Explores the relationship between one's attitudes and the way one goes through fatal illness; emphasizes forgiveness.)

Kleinman, Arthur, MD. *The Illness Narratives*. New York: Basic Books, 1988. (Exploration of the relationship between cultural metaphor and the experience of illness, focusing on Taiwanese anthropology.)

Kübler-Ross, Elisabeth, M.D. *On Death and Dying*. New York: Macmillan, 1969. (Old standard now: the first popular work that illuminated the dark specter of death.)

LeShan, Lawrence. *You Can Fight for Your Life*. New York: M. Evans & Co., 1976. (Quoting extensive research, the author links certain personality traits to cancer; stresses the importance of psychotherapy in prevention and treatment.)

Siegel, Bernie, MD. *Love, Medicine and Miracles*. New York: Harper & Row, Publishers, Inc., 1986.

_____. *Peace, Love and Healing*. New York: Harper & Row Publishers, Inc., 1989. (Balanced thinking on the relationship between attitude and the course of illness; the first articulate exploration of the disease/illness dichotomy.)

Simonton, Stephanie and Carl, M.D., and James Creighton. *Getting Well Again*. New York: Bantam Books, 1984. (Pioneering cancer and attitude book; essential reading.)

Living With Illness

Bowe, Frank. *Comeback: Six Remarkable People Who Triumphed Over Disability*. New York: Harper & Row, Publishers, Inc., 1981. (Inspirational reading for anyone who feels that his or her problem is the ultimate misery.)

Goldfarb, Lori, Mary Jane Brotherson, Jean Ann Summers, and Ann Turnbull. *Meeting the Challenge of Disability or Chronic Illness: A Family Guide*. Baltimore: Paul H. Brookes Publishing Co., 1986. (Encyclopedic help for families.)

Jewett, Claudia. *Helping Children Cope With Separation and Loss*. Boston: Harvard Common Press, 1982. (Good advice for families of seriously ill people.)

Pitzele, Sefra Kobrin. *We Are Not Alone: Learning to Live With Chronic Illness.* New York: Workman Publications, 1985. (Excellent compendium of daily practicalities and resources.)

Roach, Marion. *Another Name for Madness.* New York: Pocket Books, 1986. (Family coping with Alzheimer's disease.)

Simonton, Stephanie M. *The Healing Family.* New York: Bantam Books, 1984. (Straightforward perspectives and suggestions about issues that arise in the families of people with cancer.)

Stewart, Elizabeth. *Tangles of the Mind.* Sacramento, CA: Elderberry Press, 1991. (A daughter's adventure with her mother's Alzheimer's disease, especially her fascination with nonverbal language.)

Strong, Maggie. *Mainstay.* New York: Penguin Books, 1989. (Exploration of the caregiver's experience; essential reading for spouses of the chronically ill.)

Webster, Barbara. *All of a Piece: A Life with Multiple Sclerosis.* Baltimore: Johns Hopkins University Press, 1989. (Absorbing first-person story of a confusing, frustrating situation translatable to many chronic illnesses.)

The Doctor-Patient Relationship

Baer, Louis Shattuck, MD. *Let the Patient Decide: A Doctor's Advice to Older Persons.* Philadelphia: Westminster Press, 1978. (Practical tips for seniors who wish to have more participation in their health care.)

Inlander, Charles and Ed Weiner. *Take This Book to the Hospital With You: A Consumer Guide to Surviving Your Hospital Stay.* Emmaus, PA: Rodale Press, 1985. (Sardonic, irreverent support for patients who would really rather be home.)

Kushner, Rose. *Alternatives: New Developments in the War on Breast Cancer.* Cambridge, MA: Kensington Press, 1984. (Indomitable laywoman's crusade to limit radical mastectomies; scholarly, well-respected work.)

Mendelsohn, Robert, MD. *Confessions of a Medical Heretic.* Chicago: Contemporary Books, 1979. (Impassioned comparison of modern medicine to medieval church practices; gives the reader a broader, more skeptical perspective.)

Morra, Marion and Eve Potts. *Choices: Realistic Alternatives in Cancer Treatment.* New York: Avon Books, 1980. (Good "mainstream" information.)

Nonmedical Treatment

Hill, Ann, ed. *A Visual Encyclopedia of Unconventional Medicine.* New York: Crown Publishers, 1979. (Comprehensible and attractive introduction by reputable authorities to scores of "alternative" practices.)

The New Age Catalog. New York: Doubleday, 1988. (Guide to recent books on nonmedical practices and self-healing.)

Support Groups

Heider, John. *The Tao of Leadership.* New York: Bantam Books, 1986. (Valuable guide for leading groups with minimal intervention.)

Small, Jacquelyn. *Becoming Naturally Therapeutic.* New York: Bantam Books, 1990. (Crystal-clear guide to helping people express and understand their feelings; invaluable to support group leaders.)

Coping Skills

LeShan, Lawrence. *How To Meditate.* New York: Bantam Books, 1984. (Superb, readable meditation guide, particularly well-suited for American minds.)

McKay, Matthew, Martha Davis, and Patrick Fanning. *Messages.* Oakland, CA: New Harbinger Publications, 1983. (Excellent how-to-communicate principles and practices.)

Other New Harbinger Self-Help Titles

Men & Grief, $11.95

Lifetime Weight Control, $10.95

Acquiring Courage: An Audio Cassette Program for the Rapid Treatment of Phobias, $14.95

Getting to Sleep, $10.95

The Anxiety & Phobia Workbook, $13.95

When Once Is Not Enough: Help for Obsessive Compulsives, $11.95

Love and Renewal: A Couple's Guide to Commitment, $12.95

The Habit Control Workbook, $12.95

Love Addiction: A Guide to Emotional Independence, $11.95

The New Three Minute Meditator, $9.95

When the Bough Breaks: A Helping Guide for Parents of Sexually Abused Children, $11.95

The Relaxation & Stress Reduction Workbook, 3rd Edition, $13.95

Leader's Guide to the Relaxation & Stress Reduction Workbook, $19.95

Beyond Grief: A Guide for Recovering from the Death of a Loved One, $10.95

Thoughts & Feelings: The Art of Cognitive Stress Intervention, $12.95

Messages: The Communication Skills Book, $12.95

The Divorce Book: A Practical and Compassionate Guide, $10.95

Hypnosis for Change: A Manual of Proven Techniques, 2nd Edition, $11.95

The Deadly Diet: Recovering from Anorexia & Bulimia, $11.95

Self-Esteem, $12.95

The Better Way to Drink: Moderation and Control of Problem Drinking, $10.95

Chronic Pain Control Workbook, $13.95

Rekindling Desire: Bringing Your Sexual Relationship Back to Life, $10.95

Life Without Fear: Anxiety and Its Cure, $9.95

Visualization for Change, $12.95

Guideposts to Meaning: Discovering What Really Matters, $10.95

Controlling Stagefright: With Audiences from One to One Thousand, $10.95

Videotape: Clinical Hypnosis for Stress & Anxiety Reduction, $24.95

Starting Out Right: Essential Parenting Skills for Your Child's First Seven Years, $12.95

Big Kids: A Parent's Guide to Weight Control for Children, $10.95

Personal Peace: Transcending Your Interpersonal Limits, $10.95

My Parent's Keeper: Adult Children of the Emotionally Disturbed, $11.95

When Anger Hurts, $12.95

Free of the Shadows: Recovering from Sexual Violence, $11.95

Resolving Conflict With Others and Within Yourself, $11.95

Send a check for the titles you want, plus $2.00 for shipping and handling, to:

New Harbinger Publications, Inc.
5674 Shattuck Avenue
Oakland, CA 94609

Or write for a free catalog of all our quality self-help publications. For orders over $20 call 1-800-748-6273. Have your Visa or Mastercard number ready.